NEUROENDOCRINOLOGY AND BEHAVIOR

Edited by **Tomiki Sumiyoshi**

Neuroendocrinology and Behavior
http://dx.doi.org/10.5772/1666
Edited by Tomiki Sumiyoshi

Contributors

Jacek Kolcz, Alper Karakas, Hamit Coskun, Benjamin C. Nephew, Tomiki Sumiyoshi, Tadasu Matsuoka, Masayoshi Kurachi, Toshio Munesue, Kazumi Ashimura, Hideo Nakatani, Mitsuru Kikuchi, Shigeru Yokoyama, Manabu Oi, Haruhiro Higashida, Yoshio Minabe, Anna Tolekova, Petya Hadzhibozheva, Tsvetelin Georgiev, Stanislava Mihailova, Galina Ilieva, Maya Gulubova, Eleonora Leventieva-Necheva, Kiril Milenov, Reni Kalfin, Sihem Mbarek, Tounes Saidi, Rafika Ben Chaouacha-Chekir

Published by InTech

Janeza Trdine 9, 51000 Rijeka, Croatia

Publishing Process Manager Vedran Greblo
Technical Editor InTech DTP team
Cover InTech Design team

Additional hard copies can be obtained from orders@intechopen.com

Neuroendocrinology and Behavior, Edited by Tomiki Sumiyoshi
p. cm.
ISBN 978-953-51-0740-8

For EU product safety concerns:
IN TECH d.o.o., Prolaz Marije Krucifikse Kozulić 3, 51000 Rijeka, Croatia,
info@intechopen.com or visit our website at intechopen.com.

Meet the editor

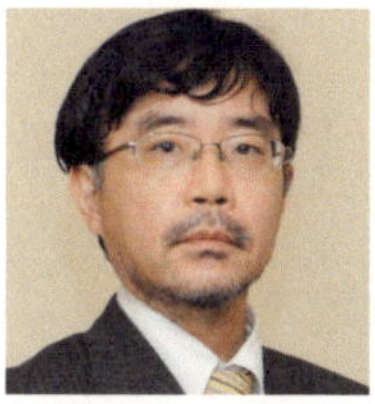

Dr Sumiyoshi obtained his MD and PhD at Kanazawa University, Japan, and is currently Clinical Professor and Director of Translational Research at the Department of Neuropsychiatry, University of Toyama Graduate School of Medicine and Pharmaceutical Sciences. He was trained at the Department of Psychiatry Case Western Reserve University as Research Associate from 1993 to 1995, and was appointed Visiting Professor in the Department of Psychiatry, Vanderbilt University from 2000 to 2002, as the founder of the augmentation pharmacotherapy to ameliorate cognitive impairment of schizophrenia. His research fields include cognitive neuroscience and psychopharmacology, as represented by more than 100 peer-reviewed articles and book chapters. Dr. Sumiyoshi is an Editorial Board member of Psychiatry Journal, and Co-Chair of Psychoneurobiology Section of World Psychiatric Association.

Contents

Preface

Understanding of the neuroendocrine system provides an insight into a wide range of bodily and mental processes, e.g. from water balance to social activity. *Neuroendocrinology and Behavior* brings its readers a concise guide to up-to-date knowledge on the function of the endocrine glands and organs in association with neurotransmitters, neuropeptides, and behavioral manifestations. In particular, this volume provides a unique medium for interactions across these multiple levels of the exploration on neuroendocrinology, behavior, and related disorders.

Various forms of stress response, e.g. anxiety and cognitive changes, have been intrinsic to both ourselves and other species. Specifically, these mechanisms involve complex interplays among physical, emotional, and behavioral processes in humans. The main concepts of this issue are reviewed in *Chapter 1* by Dr. Jacek Kolcz who also provides original data from patients suffering from acute or chronic stressors. The topics include mobilization of embryonic stem cells, as a form of stress response, during heart surgery in hospitalized patients. Drs. Alper Karakas and Hamit Coskun in *Chapter 2* report experimental studies on the regulatory role of the amygdala in learning memory. Data are presented on the effect of administration of exogenous melatonin on memory and anxiety-related behaviors in pinealectomized rats (*Part 1: The Neuroendocrine System in Cognition, Emotion, and Stress Response*).

The second part describes information on peptide hormones, i.e. oxytocin and vasopressin, and how studies of these neuropeptides enrich our understanding of social and other behaviors. In *Chapter 3,* Dr. Benjamin C. Nephew provides a review of the literature on physiological and functional roles of vasopressin and oxytocin in relation to social behaviors and mental illnesses. The need for further investigations on gender differences and stress-related mood disorders is emphasized. Drs. Tomiki Sumiyoshi, Tadasu Matsuoka, and Masayoshi Kurachi in *Chapter 4* focus on the role for the pituitary neuropeptides, particularly vasopressin, in social behavior disturbances of schizophrenia. The ability of vasopressin analogues to treat the deficits in an animal model of schizophrenia is discussed. The other pituitary neuropeptide oxytocin is currently the major focus of the therapeutic strategy for social disability of autism spectrum disorders (ASDs). Accordingly, a review on clinical trials to determine the effect of oxytocin on sociality disturbances of ASDs is provided by Drs. Toshio Munesue, Kazumi Ashimura, Hideo Nakatani, Mitsuru Kikuchi, Manabu Oi,

Haruhiro Higashida, and Yoshio Minabe in *Chapter 5* (*Part 2: Neuropeptides in Social Behaviors and Diseases*).

The functions of neuropeptides hormones also influence systemic homeostasis, e.g. modulations of smooth muscles activity, sexual behavior and reproduction, and water balance in the body. *Chapter 6* by Drs. Anna Tolekova, Petya Hadzhibozheva, Tsvetelin Georgiev, Stanislava Mihailova, Galina Ilieva, Maya Gulubova, Eleonora Leventieva-Necheva, Kiril Milenov, and Reni Kalfin presents an overview on the mechanisms of action of vasopressin, ghrelin, angiotensines, and cholecystokinins on smooth muscle organs in abdominal and pelvic cavities. The effect of cadmium, a non-essential heavy metal widely distributed in the environment, on the vasopressin system and water metabolism is investigated by Drs. Sihem Mbarek, Tounes Saidi and Rafika Ben Chaouacha-Chekir in *Chapter 7*. Exposure to cadmium was shown to modify the synthesis of vasopressin in the brain of rodents (*Part 3: Miscellaneous Issues*).

Finally, I would like to acknowledge the contributors for their excellent cooperation. I also express my gratitude to Mr. Vedran Greblo at InTech in assisting me with editing of this *Book*.

Prof. Dr. Tomiki Sumiyoshi
M.D., Ph.D., Clinical Professor and Director of Translational Research,
Department of Neuropsychiatry,
University of Toyama
Graduate School of Medicine and Pharmaceutical Sciences,
Japan

Section 1

The Neuroendocrine System in Cognition, Emotion, and Stress Response

Chapter 1

Neuroendocrine Regulation of Stress Response in Clinical Models

Jacek Kolcz

Additional information is available at the end of the chapter

http://dx.doi.org/10.5772/48533

1. Introduction

A stress response is an evolutionary heritage of ability to anticipate, identify and effectively respond to danger. After millions of years of evolution, perception of variety of stressors mobilizes neurologic, neuroendocrine, endocrine, immunologic and metabolic systems to maintain an ability to survive and propagate gens (natural selection). Additionally, in humans these mechanisms involve complex and interrelated mental, emotional, behavioral and social processes. Behavioral adaptation is aimed on modulation of neural pathways that help to cope with stressful situations. These e.g. include changes of sensory thresholds, increased alertness, memory enhancement, suppression of hunger, and stress-induced analgesia.

A stressor can be defined as a certain stimulus of the external or internal receptor. The stressors are usually divided into macroscopic threats (e.g. fight with enemy, fear, pain) and microscopic threats (targeting at epithelial or endothelial barriers e.g. infection or tissue damage). These neuroendocrine – immunologic interrelations are also vital in the clinical situations. During an acute stress response, physiological processes are aimed on redistribution of energy utilization in specific organs, inhibiting or stimulating energy mobilization. Therefore certain tissues receive sufficient supply of energy while others reduce their consumption according to priority. This is achieved mainly by: the sympathetic nervous system (SNS), release of catecholamines which inhibit insulin release and action, stimulates glucagon and ACTH production; hypothalamic – pituitary – adrenocortical (HPA) axis that in general increases gluconeogenesis and glycogenolysis, inhibits glucose uptake, and enhances proteolysis and lipolysis; hypothalamic - posterior pituitary (ADH) – kidney axis with water retention; brain – juxta-gromelular apparatus activity - (renin/ angiotensin/aldosterone - RAAS) with many effects on blood pressure, electrolytes and water balance; hypothalamic-pituitary-thyroid axis (response to cold and heat), natriuretic peptides, the parasympathetic nervous system (acetylcholine release), changes in immune system (cytokines and other pro-inflammatory substances), mediators of endothelial function and mobilization of stem cells.

In the clinical settings, variety of interesting models and complex relations can be investigated. In particular, pathophysiology and treatment of congenital heart defects create unique models of stress response. Hypoxia, circulatory insufficiency, volume or pressure overload, hypo- or hyperthermia, pain, changes in organ perfusion, disturbances of the osmolarity, inflammatory- or immune- response create exceptional milieu and environment for the research.

In this chapter we reviewed main concepts of stress response in such environment additionally presenting some results of own research. It focuses on patients who had strong stressors working in acute or chronic manner (desaturation, increased afterload, volume overload, circulatory insufficiency) with all related elements affecting the model in clinical environment.

2. The arrangement of the stress response

The stress response is the complex process that can be initiated by immune or central nervous system. The central nervous system reacts against macroscopic threats and controls whole body response. Thus, in face of lacking of the system integrity central nervous system switches all functions over to subordinate constitutive activities to defense against the threat. The hypothalamus – pituitary – adrenal axis is activated and vasopressin, prolactin and growth hormone are released. In clinical settings corticotropin realizing hormone and vasopressin (both stimulated by adreno-cortical signals e.g. pain, fear, hypovolemia or immunologic stimuli e.g. interleukins, TNF, cytokines) (1) synergistically increase adrenocorticotropin (ACTH) secretion. ACTH induces conversion of cholesterol to cortisol which cooperates with sympathetic nervous system to prepare a body for response by mobilization of energetic substrates, increase of intravascular volume and blood pressure enhancement (Tab.1.).

The immune system reacts against microscopic threats infringing endothelial or epithelial barriers. The initial signal is amplified by cascade of lymphokines and activated cells and stimulates central stress response which eventually terminates system overstimulation. Immune response and tissue damage contribute to systemic inflammatory response syndrome (SIRS) development. These inflammatory signals are transferred to the central nervous system by vagus nerve and activate HPA axis (2).

Adaptation to chronic stress in humans is not well understood and unnatural situation. It is mostly created in the clinical settings when treatment of critical disease is implemented and it reaches chronic phase. After acute stress response when ACTH, prolactin, growth hormone, and thyroid hormone are elevated, the pulsatile, more physiologic pattern of neurohormones concentration appears. Although normal limits of plasma neurohormons levels in stress response are not known, inadequate concentrations can lead to acute failure and shock.

Action	Mechanism
Growth inhibition	Decrease of DNA and RNA synthesis Increase of protein catabolism in all tissues Enhancement of protein synthesis in the liver
Substrates availability increase	Glycolysis, lipolysis, protein hydrolysis
Blood pressure increase	Vascular tone increase, Expression of adrenergic receptors Activation of renin – angiotensin – aldosterone system
Inhibition of constitutive functions	Suppression of immune response Decrease of circulating lymphocytes, monocytes and eosinophils Apoptosis induction
Anti-inflammatory	Decrease of capillary permeability, phagocytosis, leucocyte demargination, interleukine synthesis
Water balance	Sodium and water reabsorbtion

Table 1. Role of the cortisol in stress response initiation.

3. Sympathetic nervous system

Sympathetic nervous system stimulation is a part of central regulatory mechanism. It exerts many effects on the cardiovascular system by norepinephrine and epinephrine. Afferent baroreceptor signaling to the brain signals low cardiac output and efferent sympathetic pathways are activated. The main results of it are vasoconstriction (increased afterload, decreased renal perfusion), increased heart rate and contractility (increased cardiac output and wall stress), activation of RAAS. These effects are aimed on restoration of cardiac output, however, at the expense of increased myocardial oxygen demand, increased intracellular calcium toxicity, and myocardial hypertrophy. Sympathetic overstimulation can cause many undesirable effects like: expression of fetal gens, apoptosis, necrosis and remodeling and high levels of plasma norepinephrine are an independent predictor of mortality.

In clinical model of univentricular circulation characterized by increased afterload and normal saturation interesting behavioral adaptation was observed. During the exercise the heart rate at anaerobic threshold was significantly slower and patients' lung tidal volume lower compared to healthy age matched volunteers. These differences disappeared at peak effort. The effect was associated with a delayed chronotropic response of the heart and a reaction which provides a longer filling time and larger preload to the single ventricle. Delayed chronotropic response, earlier achievement of anaerobic threshold and higher value of ventilator equivalent of carbon dioxide at peak exercise obviously reflect greater impairment of cardiac output in single ventricle patients compared to healthy volunteers. The limitation of the exercise capacity is caused mainly by abnormal autonomic nervous system activity, lower non-pulsatile pulmonary flow, neurohormonal disturbances and dysfunction of the endothelium. The primary mechanism restricting exercise capacity is the lack of ability to increase and maintain the cardiac output and pulmonary flow in response to exercise. This is complementary with delayed chronotropic reaction, decreased heart rate acceleration and abnormal reflex from ergoreceptors. Exercise studies with external pacemaker heart stimulation to increase heart rate despite of slowing it reflex did not cause increase of exercise tolerance (3). In our model heart rate was significantly lower at anaerobic threshold indicating delayed chronotropic response or adaptation to the demand of increased output generation (the slower the heart rate, the better preload). This was accompanied by significant respiratory tidal volume lowering, diminished carbon dioxide production, and respiratory equivalent of carbon dioxide compared to control group. These differences disappeared at peak exercise suggesting maintenance of optimal hemodynamic and respiratory parameters for maximal physiological effect.

Effects of sympathetic stimulation	Cellular effects
Heart	Increased cardiomyocyte calcium entry
Increased contractility (inotropy)	Myocardial hypertrophy
Increased heart rate	Gene expression:
Increased wall stress	Increased expression of fetal gens
Decreased myocardial relaxation (lusitropy)	Decreased expression of calcium metabolism gens
Increased oxygen demand	Apoptosis
Peripheral vessels	Necrosis
Constriction	Fibrosis
Increased afterload	Myocardial hypertrophy / remodeling
Kidney	β1 - receptors down-regulation
Vasoconstriction	
Sodium retention	
Water retention	
RAAS activation	
Sodium retention	
Water retention	

Table 2. Sympathetic nervous system activation

Significant positive correlation of VE/VCO2 (respiratory equivalent of carbon dioxide) at peak exercise with proBNP and endothelin-1 were found. The parameter VE/VCO2 reflects relationship between minute ventilation and carbon dioxide clearance and is considered as a more sensitive prognostic factor than oxygen consumption in diagnosis of circulatory insufficiency. In patients with chronic heart failure VE/VCO2 is increased and negatively correlated with cardiac output at peak exercise and is independent of subject effort and peripheral function (3, 4). In our study VE/VCO_2 peak is significantly higher in investigated group, compared to age matched controls. The correlation with endothelin-1 and proBNP indicates the possibility of identification of such patients by neurohormonal screening tests and suggests etiology of such condition. Higher concentration of endothelin-1 reveals endothelial dysfunction and can contribute to higher resistance of pulmonary vascular bed and lower pulmonary blood flow at peak exercise. Higher BNP concentrations can indicate more pronounced ventricular dysfunction (5).

4. Hypothalamic-pituitary-adrenal axis

Hypothalamic – pitutitary – adrenal system is the central stress response system linking neural regulation to neurohormonal and humoral control. In response to cortical signals e.g. fear, pain, deep emotions or immune derived factors like TNF α, Il-6 corticotropin realizing hormone, vasopressin, prolactin and growth hormone are released. Corticotropin releasing hormone stimulates sympathetic system and ACTH secretion. It reaches the adrenal cortex and stimulates cortisol production from cholesterol. Cortisol cooperates with sympathetic activation to prepare metabolism for stress response. These mechanism inhibit all growth and developmental functions, prepare metabolic substrates (glucose, fatty acids, amino acids), increase blood pressure and intravascular volume.

There is insufficiency of hypothalamic-pituitary-adrenal axis after pediatric cardiac surgery observed, best described as a critical illness–related corticosteroid insufficiency (CIRCI). Together with other axes derangement it is considered as one of the causes of low cardiac output syndrome in postoperative period. Many causes of this phenomenon were proposed: brain hypoperfusion, central hypothalamus and pituitary gland insufficiency, tissue resistance to adrenocorticotropic hormone (ACTH), adrenal dysfunction, cyanosis and tissues immaturities.

5. Endotheline

Endothelins (ET -1,-2,-3) are a molecules produced by endothelium acting as a vasoconstrictors and mitogenic factors. In patients with heart failure their plasma concentrations are increased their concentration is proportional to the severity of the disease. Endothelins promote vasoconstriction, inflammation, fibrosis, and hypertrophy in the pulmonary and systemic vasculature.

Plasma ET-1 levels are elevated in patients who have cardiomyopathy or chronic heart failure, and correlate with severity and prognosis. In particular, the degree of plasma elevation of endothelin correlates with the magnitude of alterations in cardiac hemodynamics and functional class.

In our material, higher pulmonary artery resistance was related to higher endothelin concentration in patients with single ventricle, therefore endothelin receptor antagonist could result in reduction of pulmonary resistance.

6. Renin angiotensin aldosterone axis

Renin angiotensin aldosterone axis exerts many effects in cardiovascular system. Neural connexion of the brain and kidneys is stimulated by low sodium, decreased perfusion, increased alpha – adrenergic activity. It can effect juxtaglomerular apparatus increasing renien - protease transforming angiotensinogen to angiotensin I which is converted within the endothelial cells (particularly concentrated in the lungs) to angiotensin II by angiotensin-converting enzyme (ACE). Angiotensin II is the most potent vasoconstrictor increasing vascular resistance in stress situations (especially in hypovolemia) and effecting adrenal cortex increasing aldosterone production which increases reclaiming of sodium and water. And its major role is to maintain the circulating volume status.

7. Vasopressin system

Vasopressin (ADH) is released by the hypothalamus as a result of baroreceptor, osmotic, and neurohormonal stimuli. It normally maintains body fluid balance, vascular tone, and regulates contractility. Heart failure causes a paradoxical increase in AVP. The increased blood volume and atrial pressure in heart failure suggest inhibition of vasopressin secretion, but it does not occur. This phenomenon is related to SNS and RAAS activation overriding the volume and low-pressure cardiovascular receptors and osmotic vasopressin regulation causing increase in AVP secretion. It contributes to the increased systemic vascular resistance (V1 receptors) and to renal retention of fluid (V2 receptors). Stimulation of V1 receptors can also case vasoconstriction of the peripheral vessels, platelet aggregation, and adrenocorticotrophic hormone stimulation. Low-dose arginine infusion initiated in the operating room after complex neonatal cardiac surgery was associated with decreased fluid resuscitation and catecholamine. The vasopressin levels are usually high in the early phase of septic shock, but it's deficiency was noted in vasodilatory shock.

The important mechanism of vasopressin action in stress states is its potentiating effect on ACTH secretion leading to cortisol release. Although vasopressin is a powerful vasoconstrictor it dilates the pulmonary, cerebral, and myocardial circulations helping to preserve vital organ blood flow.

In our group of patients with single ventricle, there was a significant correlation between vasopressin concentration and disturbances of water – electrolyte balance in single ventricle patients. Higher vasopressin plasma levels were connected with greater propensity for fluid retention and prolonged pleural effusions (6).

8. Thyroid hormones

Thyroid hormones are stimulated by TSH anterior pituitary secretion. There is many actions of thyroid hormones on cardiovascular system exerted mainly by triiodothyronine (T3). These effects can be divided into genomic and extragenomic actions. T3 bounds to the nuclear receptors and activates many gens corresponding to key myocardial functions: myosin heavy chain (MHC), sarcoplasmic reticulum Caţţ-ATPase (SERCA2) and its inhibitor phospholamban (affecting cardiac contractile function and diastolic relaxation), voltage-gated Kţ channels, b1-adrenergic receptor, guanine nucleotide regulatory proteins, adenylate cyclase, NAţ/Kţ-ATPase, and Na/Ca exchanger. The main cardiovascular effects of T3 are: increased cardiac contractility, reduction of afterload, reduction of vascular resistance, chronotropic effect (increased heart rate), increases sodium reabsorption and water improves atrial filing pressure. All of this increase cardiac output.

T3 has genomic effects that maintain endothelial integrity, such as angiotensin receptors in vascular smooth muscle cells (VSMC). This supports the hypothesis that the vasculature is a principal target for T3 action. T3 decreases resistance in peripheral arterioles. Extragenomic actions include: modulation of cellular metabolic activities, such as glucose and amino acid transport, ion fluxes at the level of the plasma membrane, and mitochondrial gene expression and function.

9. Cholinergic pathway

Together with the stimulation of the adrenergic system the feedback is also started as anti-inflammatory cholinergic pathway. It is comprised of vagus nerve signals leading to acetylcholine interaction with receptors on monocytes and macrophages, resulting in reduced cytokine production. It can prevent tissue injury and improve survival by external stimulation. The cholinergic anti-inflammatory pathway exerts a tonic, inhibitory influence on immune responses to infection and tissue injury. Interrupting this pathway, produces exaggerated responses to bacterial products and injury.

10. Natruretic peptydes

Natruretic peptide system counteracts of some of the effects of neurohormonal activation causing vasodilatation, reduction of aldosterone production (by direct influence on the adrenal gland), increased diuresis and natriuresis, reduction of renin production, decreased vasopressin realize, decreased activation of the sympathethic nervous system. Direct influence of the naturetic peptydes on the myocardium includes prevention of hypertrophy and reduction of fibroblast proliferation. BNP is a natriuretic peptide released in response to ventricular volume expansion and pressure overload.

Cardiopulmonary by-pass in children induces renal and neurohormonal changes similar to those observed in congestive heart failure: upregulation of the RAA axis, increase of renin concentration, release of vasopressin. The endogenous biological activity of natriuretic hormone system is decreased after the bypass. This is caused by deficiency of biologically active neurohormons, presence of inactive neurohormons, resistance to natriuretic hormone activity, receptor down-regulation, abnormal signal transduction, increased phosphodiesterase activity.

It has been also shown that neurohormons can decrease ischemia-reperfusion injury in multiple tissue including heart by inhibition of angiotensin II and aldosterone, limitation of intracellular Ca^{++} overload, maintainance of ATP stores, preservation of myofibril, mitochondrial and nuclear structure of cardiomyocytes.

In the natural history of diseased cardiovascular system complex interactions between local, humoral, and neural factors lead to abnormalities in the circulatory control. These adaptive responses are aimed at maintaining adequate vital organ perfusion but can lead to unfavorable and undesirable changes both in the heart and the vascular system. An impaired regulation of cardiac autonomic system and activation of many neurohormonal factors as well as the rennin-angiotensin-aldosterone system (RAAS). These changes may contribute to numerous early and late complications e.g. dysregulation of fluid homeostasis, effusions, detrimental remodeling, protein-losing enteropathy and limited exercise capacity. They can also serve as important indices for risk stratification, prediction of unfavorable events and adjustment of treatment (3).

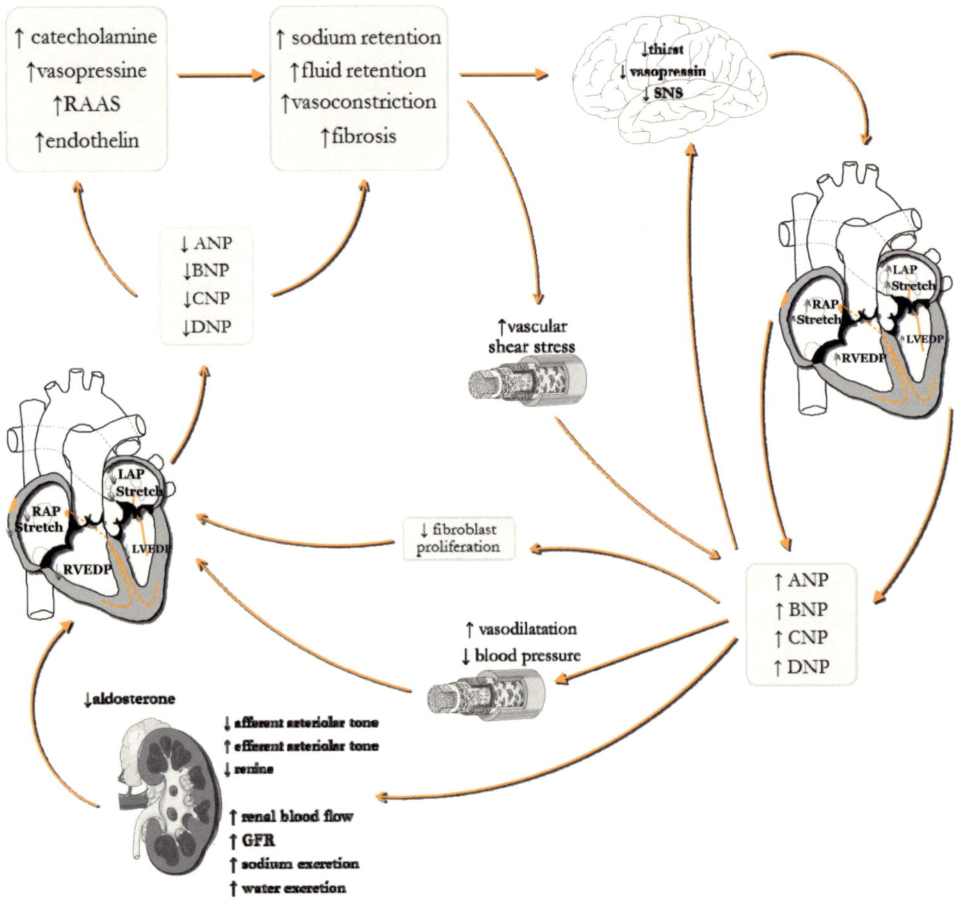

Figure 1. Natruretic factors interactions.

11. Stem cells

Stem cells are specific cells with ability to unlimited divisions and differentiation. There are many types of stem cells depending on the differentiation degree. Residual small cells with embryonic stem cells phenotype (*VSELs, Very Small Embryonic-like Cells*) are a population of pluripotent cells deposited in developing organs during embryogenesis. In the bone marrow

VSELs find beneficial conditions to growth and become reserve cell line participating in tissue and organ regeneration. In the postnatal life they are inactive and flow in blood stream in small amount. Mobilization of VSEL's is considered as a part of stress response it can increase upon different impulses e.g. tissue damage, ischemia, hypoxia, myocardial infarction, open heart surgery, extracorporeal circulation. Cells mobilized from bone marrow penetrate to blood and are attracted to damaged tissues by chemotactic factors, e.g. SDF-l, HGF/SF, or VSEGF.

Researches who identified and described morphology of VSELs also showed the ability of those cells to proliferate and differentiate into all three primary germ layers in appropriate differentiating medium. It has been also proved that VSELs express many markers of primordial germ cells, e.g. fetal alkaline phosphatase, Oct-4, SSEA-l, CXCR4, Mvh, Stella, Fragilis, Nobox and Hdac6, indicating their similarity to germ cells through which genes are passed from generation to generation – the best reservoir of stem cells (7, 8). Most active translocation of stem cells takes place during early stage of human embryogenesis. In the beginning of gastrulation and organogenesis stem cells migrate to places of new tissues and organs formation. Subsequently, stem cells settle down in tissue specific spaces and constitute a cell line undergoing self-renewal process. These cells also replenish damaged or apoptotic cells during individual life. VSELs may accumulate in bone marrow under the influence of chemotactic factors (correlation between CXCR4 receptor and lymphokine SDF-1). After colonizing bone marrow VSELs find beneficial conditions to growth and become reserve cell line participating in tissue and organ regeneration. In normal conditions VSELs circulate in the peripheral blood in small number and can increase upon different stimuli e.g. tissue damage or severe stress (ischemia, hypoxia, myocardial infarction, open heart surgery, extracorporeal circulation) (9). Cells mobilized from bone marrow penetrate to blood and are attracted to damaged tissues by chemotactic factors, e.g. SDF-l, HGF/SF, or VSEGF. It has been proved that many clinical scenarios are associated with increase of stem cells in bloodstream. Increase of the number of bone marrow derived stem cells was observed in skeletal muscle injury, myocardial infarction, stroke, bones fractures, leasions of the liver and kidneys, ischaemia of the extremities and after lung or liver transplantation. These cells were described as endothelial progenitor cells (EPC), myocardial or muscle progenitor cells, neural progenitor cells, liver progenitor cells etc… These data indicate that during injury of the tissues and organs non-hematopoetic stem cells are mobilized from the marrow (10) and probably from other tissue niches to the blood where they circulate as a source of the stem cells supporting regeneration of the tissues (11, 12). This process is governed by injured tissue derived chemoattractants such as SDF-l, and other factors e.g.: VEGF, HGF/SF, UF and FGF-2. It is also known that transcriptional factor HIF-1 (hypoxia regulated/induced transcription factor) connected with the tissue ischemia takes important palce in regulation of expression of these factors. The promotor for sdf-l, vegf and hgf/sf gens have bounding places for HIF-1. Therefore hypoxia / cyanosis can induce expression of factors responsible for stem cells releasing and their migration to the injured tissues and organs. VSELs which are present in the marrow are quiescent and they need unknown factors for activation and stimulation of their activity. These incentives and modulators are unknown.

Recent research indicates that in the mature hearts of the mammalians there is a population of the cells capable of mitotic divisions named cardiac stem cells (CSC). They are pluripotential, clonogenic, and self-replicable. Their location in the herat seems to be related to the mechanical load of given segment of the heart muscle and is inversely proportional to hemodynamic load. The number of CSC depends on the methodology of counting and ranges from 1/8000 to 1/20 000 cardiomyocytes or 1/ 32 000 – 1/80 000 all cells of the heart.

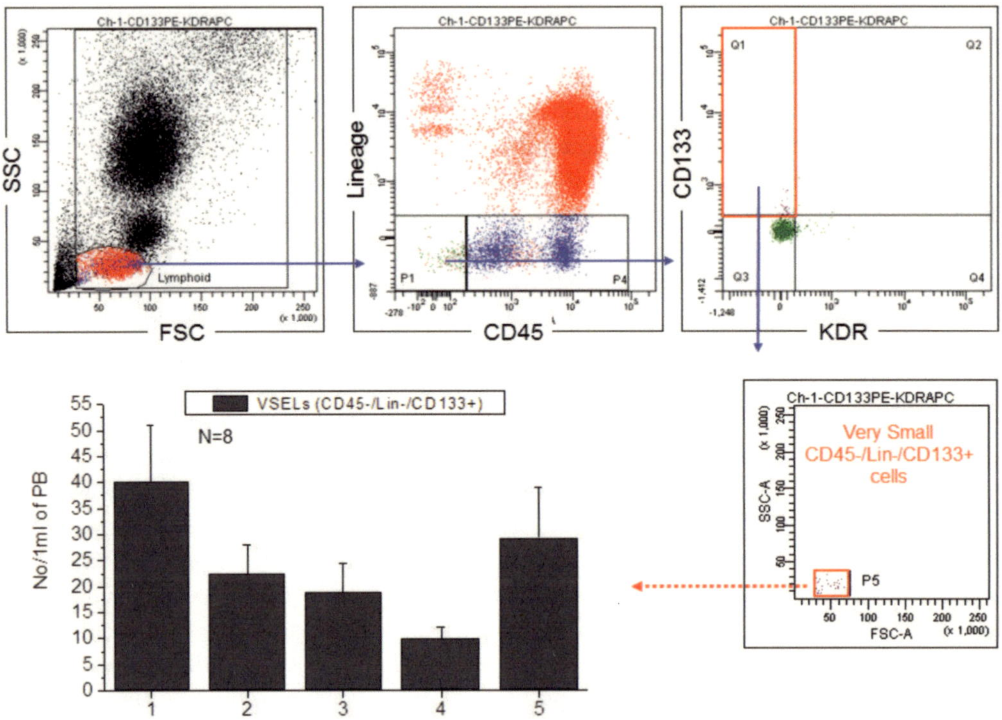

Figure 2. Flow cytometry – mobilization of VSELs in children undergoing heart surgery due to congenital heart diseases

In population of our patients we've obtained blood specimens before the operation and during the hospitalization to determine the level of VSELs mobilization. Using the flow cytometry it has been shown that VSELs appears in peripheral blood with a specified pattern of mobilization during surgery and directly after it (Fig.2.) and confirmed the presence of those cells within myocardium Fig.3.

The acute phase of stress response is characterized by increased release of neuroendocrine mediators from the hypothalamus and pituitary. This is aimed on the blood pressure maintenance and mobilization of fuel substrates at the expense of deregulation of homeostatic mechanisms, immunologic response, growth, development and regeneration. If stress response is insufficient to maintain tissue perfusion, shock appears.

During the prolonged phase of critical illness, the effects of the stress response mediators, may be harmful. Decreased levels of anterior pituitary hormones and loss of the normal pattern of pulsatile release of these hormones characterize the prolonged phase of critical illness. Cortisol levels remain elevated in chronic critical illness despite a decrease in ACTH release. The metabolic result of this neuroendocrine array is worsen metabolism of fatty acids and a propensity for fat storing and protein wasting. The immune effects related to neuroendocrine disturbances are impaired lymphocyte and monocyte function and increased lymphocyte apoptosis. It leads to catabolic state and multiple organ dysfunction. Duration of immune suppression correlates strongly with the incidence of related infection. Tissue damage and strong stressors (such as cyanosis, circulatory insufficiency) stimulate regenerative and reparative processes involving stem cells.

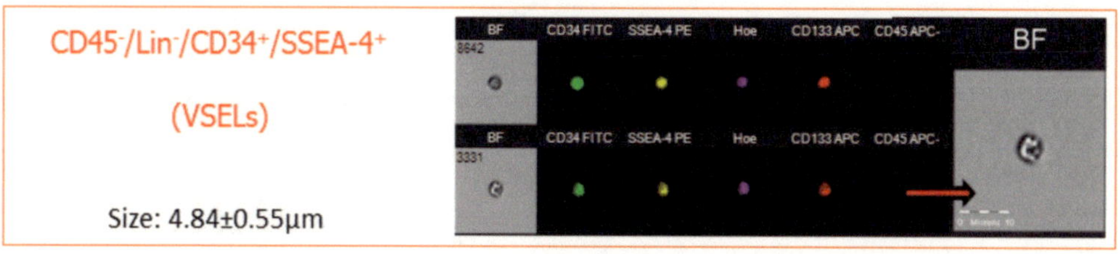

Figure 3. Very small embryonic-like cells extracted from the heart

Author details

Jacek Kolcz
Department of Pediatric Cardiac Surgery, Polish - American Children's Hospital, Jagiellonian University, Krakow, Poland

Acknowledgement

This work is supportet by government grant No 2011/01/B/NZ5/04246

12. References

[1] Chesnokova V, Melmed S. Endocrinology. Neuro-immuno-endocrine modulation of the hypothalamic-pituitary-adrenal (HPA) axis by gp130 signaling molecules. 2002 May;143(5):1571-4.

[2] Johnston GR, Webster NR Cytokines and the immunomodulatory function of the vagus nerve. Br J Anaesth. 2009 Apr;102(4):453-62.

[3] Francis DP, Shamim W, Davies LC, Piepoli MF, Ponikowski P, Anker SD, Coats AJ. Cardiopulmonary exercise testing for prognosis in chronic heart failure: continuous and independent prognostic value from VE/VCO(2)slope and peak VO(2). Eur Heart J 2000;21:154–161.

[4] Arena R, Humphrey R. Comparison of ventilatory expired gas parameters used to predict hospitalization in patients with heart failure. Am Heart J 2002;143:427–432.

[5] Koch AM, Zink S, Singer H, Dittrich S. B-type natriuretic peptide levels in patients with functionally univentricular hearts after total cavopulmonary connection. Eur J Heart Fail 2008;10:60–62.

[6] Kolcz J, Tomkiewicz-Pajak L, Wojcik E, Podolec P, Skalski J. Prognostic significance and correlations of neurohumoral factors in early and late postoperative period after Fontan procedure. Interact Cardiovasc Thorac Surg. 2011 Jul;13(1):40-5.

[7] Kucia M, Wu W, Ratajczak MZ Bone marrow-derived very smali embryonic like stem cells (VSEL) – their developmental origin and biologica/ signijicance. Deve/op. Dynamics 2007,236:3309-3320.

[8] Kucia M, Zuba-Surma E, Wysoczynski M, Wu W, Ratajczak J, Ratajczak MZ Adult marrow-derived vety small embryonic-like stem cells (VSEL SC) and tissue engineering Exp. Opinion Biol. Ther. 2007, 499-514.

[9] Wojakowski W, Tendera M, Kucia M, Zuba-SurmaE, Paczkowska E, Ciosek J, Ha/asa M, Król M, Kaźmierski ,Ocha A, Ratajczak J, Machaliński B, Ratajczak MZ Mobilization of Bone Marrow-Derived Oct-4+SSEA-4+ Vely Smali Embryonic-Like Stem Cells in Patients with Acute myocardial infarction . J Am Col Cardiol. 20.09,53, 1-9

[10] Kucia M, Wysoczynski M, Wan W, Zuba-Surma EK, Ratajczak J, Ratajczak MZ Evidence that very small embryonic like (VSEL) stemcells are mobilized intoperipheral blood. StemCells 20.0.8,26,20.83-20.92

[11] Kucia M, Ratajczak J, Ratajczak MZ. Bone Marrew as a SOUlU oj Circulating CXCR4 Tissue Commilled Stem Cells (TCSC). Bio!. Celi 2005,97, 133-/46.

[12] Kucia M, Dawn D, Hunt C, Wysoczynski M, Majka M, Ratajczak 1, Rezzoug F. lldstad ST, Bolli R, Ratajczak M.Z Cells expressing markers of cardiac tissue-committedstemcells reside in the bonemarrow and are mobilized into peripheral bloodfollowing myocardial infraction. Cir Research 20.04, 95, 1191- 1199.

Chapter 2

Intraamygdalar Melatonin Administration and Pinealectomy Affect Anxiety Like Behavior and Spatial Memory

Alper Karakas and Hamit Coskun

Additional information is available at the end of the chapter

http://dx.doi.org/10.5772/48690

1. Introduction

1.1.The pineal gland

The pineal gland, which is called as "seat of the rational soul" by Descartes, is a pine shaped, unpaired organ located at the epithalamus of the brain. The invagination of the diencephalon develops the pineal gland and it is connected to the habenular commissure with a stalk. There is a close link between the pineal gland and the third ventricle of the brain and the area of the third ventricle receiving the pineal stalk is known as the pineal recess. The pineal gland has an endogenous, circadian(around 24 hours) rhythmic pattern in its metabolic and/or neural activity. The weight and the volume of the pineal gland show big differences within and between the species depending on the time of year, age and the physiological status of the animal. The volume of the pineal gland tends to increase in line with increasing body weight (Binkley, 1988).

The mammalian pineal is specialized for only secretion whereas fish and amphibian pineal glands acting as a photoreceptive organ and in reptiles and in birds, pineal gland is both receiving the light and has secretory function. In some birds and lower vertebrates, pineal gland also works as a rhythm generator but in mammals it is working in the coordination of rhythm physiology. In mammals, the rhythm generator is located in the suprachiasmatic nuclei of the hypothalamus (Refinetti et al, 1994). Some fish, amphibians and reptiles have a pineal gland with the two components, namely, the extracranial parietal organ and the intracranial pineal organ (Arendt, 1995).

The neuronal innervation of the pineal gland in lower vertebrates and mammals is not alike because of the lost of the efferent innervation during the phylogenesis in lower vertebrates.

The post-ganglionic sympathetic fibers arising from the superior cervical ganglion innervates mainly pineal gland of the mammals. Postganglionic fibers reaching the pineal organ via the nervi conarii release norepinephrine at night. This neurotransmitter then activates adenylate cyclase, stimulating production of the second messenger cyclic adenosine monophosphate (cAMP), which accelerates melatonin synthesis. The vascular supply of the pineal gland is very rich. The arterial supply of the pineal gland is provided by the branches of the posterior choroidal arteries. There is also a well-developed internal capillary network in pineal gland (Quay, 1974).

1.2. Melatonin hormone

1.2.1. General information about melatonin hormone

Melatonin was first identified by Lerner and colleagues in 1958, as the constituent of bovine pineal glands that lightens isolated frog skin. After it's discovery, many studies focused on the physiologic roles of melatonin on pigmentation in lower vertebrates and gonodal maturation in mammals.

Pineal gland functions as a chemical neurotransducer which converts the neural stimuli to a hormonal product as melatonin. This gland regulates many physiological functions by secreting and releasing melatonin. In the secretion of melatonin, the time of the day, age of the animal and in some photoperiodic species, time of year may be important determinant. Melatonin is secreted and released in a circadian fashion, high levels at night and very low levels at day time (Arendt, 1988). The circadian rhythm of melatonin release persists in constant darkness. However, this rhythm can be altered by nighttime light exposure, because light can suppress melatonin production. Many physiological rhythms are synchronized by the normal daily variations of the melatonin secretion. The nighttime sleep initiation and maintenance in diurnal species is also controlled by the melatonin secretion.

Light information is first received by the retina of the eye. This information is transferred to Suprachiasmatic nuclei (SCN) by the retinohypothalamic tract. SCN is capable of measuring the length of the dark/light. The information of light is then transferred to Superior Cervical Ganglia (SCG) of the spinal cord. Pineal gland receives the projections from postganglionic sympathetic nerve endings emerging from the SCG which release norepinephrine (NE). The secretion of melatonin determined by the NE since the release of NE is associated with darkness. In as much as NE release onto the pinealocytes occurs at night, melatonin synthesis likewise occurs primarily during darkness. Therefore, the concentration of melatonin in the blood is greater at night than during the day. Some other factors such as the species and tissues may influence the rate and the pattern of the nocturnal increase in melatonin production (Sugden, 1991; Klein, 1993).

Melatonin has a half life of nearly 20-40 minutes. It does not remain in the blood very long. Unless the pineal gland continues to produce and secrete melatonin, blood levels of the hormone drop quickly. Melatonin is removed from the blood in at least four ways. 1) It is enzymatically degraded primarly to 6-hydroxy melatonin by the liver. 2) Melatonin that is taken up by other cells is non enzymatical degraded when it scavenges hydroxyl radicals. 3) Also, melatonin in the blood rapidly escapes into other body fluids. 4) Finally, melatonin attaches to specific receptors or binding sites located at various locations in the organism (Panke et al, 1979; Steinlechner, 1996).

The melatonin receptors involved in mediating the effects of melatonin on the reproductive and endocrine systems are presumed to be those located in the pars tuberalis of the anterior pituitary gland (Stankov et al, 1991). These cells are in close proximity to the primary portal plexus and the terminals of the hypothalamic releasing hormone neurosecretory cells in the median eminence. Melatonin theoretically controls the release of substances, e.g., gonadotropins or other factors, that act in a paracrine manner in the nearby median eminence thereby regulating the release of the hypothalamic releasing hormones, e.g., gonadotropin releasing hormone (GnRH). In this manner melatonin can obviously regulate the functional status of the gonads and control the reproductive capability of an animal on a seasonal basis.

Melatonin modulates many physiological functions such as sleep, circadian, visual, cerebrovascular, reproductive, neuroendocrine, and neuroimmunological functions (Arendt, 2000; Wirz-Justice, 2001; Borjigin et al., 1999; Brzezinzki, 1997; Masana and Dubocovich, 2001; Vanecek, 1999; Hardeland et al., 2006). The amphilicity of the melatonin is allowing the molecule to enter any cell, compartment or body fluid (Poeggeler et al., 1994). In addition to physiological functions, melatonin influences the behavioural processes such as learning, stress, anxiety like behaviors, and depression (Krause and Dubocovich, 1990; Mantovani et al, 2003; Naranjo-Rodriguez et al., 2000; Loiseau et al., 2006). With regard to behavioural processes, melatonin binding sites have been found in the regions implicated in cognition and memory in the brain (Cardinalli et al., 1979; Weaver et al., 1989). The previous studies have shown that passive and active avoidance learning are affected by melatonin (Martini, 1971; Kovács et al., 1974). Melatonin that decreases recognition time, leads to a facilitation of short-term memory (Argyriou et al, 1998]. Taken together, these findings suggest the beneficial effect of melatonin on cognition and memory.

Melatonin receptors represent saturation by the melatonin concentrations, which are close to physiologic nighttime melatonin levels. Because of this reason, these receptors show a dosage dependent activity. The sleep-promoting and activity-inhibiting effects of melatonin are provided by its low levels (e.g.,50 pg/mL in blood plasma) at the beginning of the night. However, the high levels of melatonin (e.g.,150 pg/mL in blood plasma) do not enhance these behavioral parameters. Some diurnal variations are also evident in the sensitivity of the melatonin receptors since melatonin receptors are more sensitive during the daytime when the time endogenous melatonin is not secreted. The circadian phase shifting effect of melatonin may be due to the enhanced sensitivity of melatonin receptors to melatonin in the morning or in the evening hours in response to small increases in melatonin secretion (Reppert, 1997).

1.2.2. The role of melatonin hormone on anxiety and learning performance

Melatonin seems to produce anxiolytic (Naranjo-Rodriguez et al., 2000; Papp et al., 2000) effects. The effect of melatonin on anxiety is suggested to be mediated by central gamma amino butyric acid (GABA) neurotransmission (Golombek et al., 1996). The literature findings have provided evidence for an interaction between melatonin and central GABA neurotransmission. GABA release is augmented by melatonin in rat brain tissue *in vitro* (Niles et al., 1987; Coloma and Niles, 1988). Also, when melatonin was applied *in vivo*, GABA levels increased in several brain regions in rats (Rosenstein and Cardinali, 1986; Xu et al., 1995). These findings mean that melatonin increases GABA levels, which in turn may affect anxiety of animals.

It has been shown that melatonin affects passive and active avoidance learning. Melatonin that decreases recognition time, leads to a facilitation of short-term memory. We have previously shown that melatonin implementations have some effects on learning performance depending on treatment. We investigated the effects of pinealectomy, constant release melatonin implants, and timed melatonin injections on spatial memory in male rats by using Morris water maze. Our findings showed that spatial memory performance of the rats was impaired by the pinealectomy and melatonin injections since they elongated the latency and shortened the time passed in the correct quadrant. Melatonin implantation did not change significantly the spatial memory performance of the rats. This outcome suggests that while the removal of the pineal gland and exogenous administration of melatonin via injections did impair learning performance, constant release melatonin administration via implantation did not affect the spatial memory in Wistar albino rats. There is also consistent research evidence that melatonin given from weaning did lead to learning and memory deficit in rats (Cao et al., 2009). Despite this new emerging evidence in the literature, there is more research needed for illuminating the role of the implementations on the various areas of the rat's brain. For instance, the effect of intraamygdalar melatonin administration on anxiety-like behaviors and spatial learning has not been investigated yet.

1.2.3. Pinealectomy

Pinealectomy is one of the methods to investigate the effect of melatonin in animals. It eliminates the melatonin hormone from blood circulation. It is well-recognized that the removal of the pineal gland abolishes the rhythmic endogenous melatonin release and decreases the plasma levels of melatonin significantly (Hoffman and Reiter, 1965). It prevents the animal from responding against the changes in day length (Hoffmann and Reiter, 1965; Hoffmann, 1974).

The effects of pinealectomy have been mostly studied on the reproductive system. The reproductive cycle desynchronizes from the environmental photoperiodic cycle by the pinealectomy. The effects of pinealectomy on reproductive system have been well documented in some hamster species. Pinealectomy prevents the regression effect of short photoperiods while gonadal maintenance on long photoperiods is not affected in Syrian hamster (Hoffmann and Reiter, 1965). Pinealectomy blocks short photoperiod induced gonadal regression of hamsters previously housed on long photoperiod (Hoffmann, 1974).

In addition to studies on the effects of regulatory function of pinealectomy on the reproductive system, it has been received a research attention in the behavioral studies.

However, these studies have provided rather inconsistent findings. For instance, while the pinealectomy itself did not have a detrimental effect on cognitive performance in rats, the interaction of it with the other lesion (i.,e, lesion on habenula) impaired such performance (Lecourtier et al., 2005). Many studies have shown that pinealectomy did not have a significant effect on the acquisition and extinction of the active avoidance behavior (Appenrodt and Schwarzberg, 2003), anxiety behavior (Appenrodt and Schwarzberg, 2000), passive avoidance learning (Appenrodt and Schwarzberg, 1999), open field exploratory activity (Kovács et al., 1974), and social recognition (Appenrodt et al., 2002).

1.3. The amygdala regulate the behaviours related to the anxiety and memory

In this section, the general features of the amygdala and its role on anxiety like behaviors and learning performance will be examined.

1.3.1. General features of amygdala

The amygdala, a complex mass of gray matter, is located within the anterior-medial portion of the temporal lobe, just rostral to the hippocampus. The subnuclei and cortical regions of the amygdala are connected to other nearby cortical areas on the ventral and medial aspect of the hemispheric surface. The amygdala has three major functional and anatomical subdivisions, each of which are connected to the other parts of the brain. The first subdivision, namely the medial group of subnuclei, is connected to the olfactory bulb and the olfactory cortex. The second one, the basal-lateral group, has major projections with the cerebral cortex. The third one, the central and anterior group of nuclei, makes connections with the hypothalamus and brainstem which process sensory information with hypothalamic and brainstem effector systems. The visual, somatic sensory, visceral sensory, and auditory stimuli information are provided by the cortical inputs. The amygdala and the hypothalamus are separated from each other by the pathways from sensory cortical areas (Gilman and Newman, 1992.

The amygdala receives some projections directly from thalamic nuclei, the olfactory bulb, and visceral sensory relays in the brainstem. There is evidence for this convergence of sensory information. For instance, many neurons in the amygdala are sensitive to visual, auditory, somatic, sensory, visceral sensory, gustatory, and olfactory stimuli. In addition to sensory inputs, the prefrontal and temporal cortical connections of the amygdala also make connections with cognitive neocortical circuits or integrative areas, especially for integration of the emotional significance of sensory stimuli with guide complex behavior, or vice versa. Moreover, projections from the amygdala to the hypothalamus and brainstem involve in the processing of emotions such as fear, anger, and pleasure (Gilman and Newman, 1992).

1.3.2. The role of amygdala on anxiety like behavior and learning performance

It has been demonstrated that amygdala plays a regulatory role for behaviors related to anxiety and depression (Hale et al., 2006; Blackshear et al., 2007; Martinez et al., 2007). Serotonergic activity is especially high in amygdala (Abrams et al., 2004 a, 2004b). For instance, a research has indicated that mCPP (a serotonin receptor agonist) microinjections to amygdala increased behavioral indices of anxiety without altering general activity level. In other words, it decreased open arm time and entries, but increased the closed arm ones (Cornelio and Nunes de Souza, 2007). In another study, Herdade et al. (2006) injected locally muscimol (a $GABA_A$ receptor agonist) to the medial nucleus of the amygdala and found that such treatment inhibited escape behavior in elevated T maze.

In addition to the regulatory role of amygdala in anxiety, amygdala is of great importance in regulating memory and learning functions. The amygdala is responsible for determining what memories are stored and where the memories are stored in the brain. The removal of the temporal lobe in animals leads to an impairment in memory and this impairment is global and thus none of the sensory memory is developed. For instance, the subjects experience difficulties in learning new material (i.e., anterograde amnesia) after the removal of amygdala (Almonte et al., 2007). One research has shown that amygdala damage leads to an impairment of learning an association between an auditory cue and food reward. When scopolamine, the muscarinic receptor antagonist, was injected to amygdala, it impaired performance on conditioned place preference task but not a spatial radial maze task (McIntyre et al., 1998). Moreover, the infusion of nicotinic receptor antagonists methyllycaconitine (MLA) or dihydro-b-erythroidine (DHbE) impaired working memory (Addy et al., 2003). Taken together, these findings suggest that amygdala damage has detrimental effect on the cognitive performance. However, the effect of melatonin administration to amygdala was not well known prior to the research mentioned below. The administration of melatonin to amygdala with the abolishment of melatonin hormone via pinealectomy might produce different effects on anxiety-like and learning behaviors. In other words, the endogeneous melatonin concentration and the rhythm of melatonin release might affect the effects of exogeneous melatonin administration on such behaviors.

2. Materials and methods

2.1. Animal care

A total of forty seven adult male Wistar rats (200 – 250 g) were obtained from our laboratory colony maintained at the Abant Izzet Baysal University (AIBU). They were exposed from birth to 12L (12 hour of light, 12 hour of darkness, lights off at 1800 hr). Animals were maintained in plastic cages (16x31x42 cm) with pine shavings used as bedding. Food pellets and tap water were accessible ad libitum. The procedures in this study were carried out in accordance with the Animal Scientific procedure and approved by the Institutional Animal Care and Use Committee. All lighting was provided by the cool-white fluorescent tubes controlled by automatic programmable timers. The ambient temperatures in the animal facilities were held constant at 22 ± 2 °C in air-ventilated rooms.

2.2. Experimental protocol

A total of the forty seven male adult rats were used and were randomly divided into two groups as control (sham –pinealectomy) and pinealectomy in this study. In the control group, animals were exposed to the same surgical procedure with the experimental group except for the removal of the pineal gland. We performed the four subgroups as Melatonin (1 and 100 μg/kg) (n:14), Saline (0.9%NaCl) (n:5) and Diazepam (2mg/kg) (n:5) under control and pinealectomy groups. All pinealectomies and cannulation surgeries were applied before starting the experiment. The experiments were started after a week of the pinealectomies and implantations, when surgery wounds healed up completely. The anxiety-like behaviour of animals were tested by open field and elevated plus maze tests, and spatial memory was tested by means of the Morris water maze test. All animals were exposed to these behavioral tests after 30 minutes of melatonin, saline, and diazepam administrations.

2.3. Anesthesia

Before surgery, rats were anesthetized subcutaneously with Ketamine (20 mg/kg BW, Sigma Chemical Company, MO, USA) and intraperiotoneally with pentobarbitol (32.5 mg/kg BW). The depth of anesthesia was monitored by frequent testing for the presence of leg flexion reflexes and active muscle tonus. After awaking from anesthesia, the animals were placed in their cages.

2.4. Cannulation

Cannula was implanted into the amygdala. The rats were anesthetized and fixed in a stereotaxic instrument (Stoelting Co., IL, USA) and a hole was opened at the skull by a dental drill; a 22-gauge stainless steel guide cannula 313-G/Spc (Plastics One Inc., VA, USA) was implanted aseptically into amygdala region (coordinates: - 2.6 mm posterior to the bregma; + 4.3 mm lateral to the midline and -8.4 mm ventral according to the skull). The guide cannula was secured in place by dental cement (Dental Products of Turkey, Istanbul) affixed to two mounting screws. A stainless steel dummy cannula was used to occlude the guide cannula when not in use. Each cannulated rat was then kept individually for a week to recover from surgery.

2.5. Pinealectomy

The pinealectomy of Wistar rats was performed according to the method of Hoffmann and Reiter [26]; aspiration was used to control the hemorraging. The anesthetized rats were placed in a stereotaxic apparatus to stabilize the head during surgery. After the head was shaved the surgical area was sterilized with 70% ethanol, an incision was made in the scalp. Muscle attachments were removed from the dorsal skull. After drying the skull, an incomplete circular cut was made with a dental drill burr at the λ (lambda) suture and a piece of cranium covering the pineal gland was folded forward anteriorly. The fine-tipped forceps were used to extend into the confluence of the sinuses to grasp and remove the pineal gland. After the removal of the pineal gland, the bone flap was replaced and a small square of absorbable gelatin sponge (Gelfoam, Up John, Kalamazoo, MI) was applied to the skull surface to help promote clotting. The scalp was closed with stainless steel surgical clips. After the surgery, the incision was treated with Newskin adhesive to prevent any contamination. At the end of the experiment, pinealectomized animals were decapitated and checked for the security of the pinealectomy.

2.6. Melatonin administrations

First, melatonin was dissolved in 100% ethanol (1/10 μl) and then diluted in saline (0.9 % NaCl) (9/10 μl) to the desired concentrations. Stock solutions were kept at 4 °C prior to use. The stock was diluted with sterile saline to the desired concentrations in order to make fresh working melatonin solutions. Vehicle solutions were made in the ratio of one part absolute ethanol to 1000 parts sterile saline. Melatonin was injected in a dose of either 1 or 100 μg/kg (15:00 pm).

2.7. Open field

Open-field test was taken place in a 80 cm×80 cm arena with 40 cm high walls. The open field has been the most widely used test in animal psychology. In this test, an animal (usually a rodent) is introduced into a plain and illuminated arena and its behavior is commonly regarded as a fundamental index of general behavior. In this experiment a video camera (Gkb CC-28905S, Commat LTD.ŞTİ. Ankara/Turkey) was mounted above the arena, recording behavior into the *Ethovision* videotracking system (Noldus Ethovision, Version 6, Netherland; Commat LTD.ŞTİ. Ankara/Turkey) that provided a variety of behavioral measures including distance, time in the edge, time in the center, frequency in the edge, frequency in the center, mobility and velocity among the different areas of the arena. All animals were then returned to the breeding and exhibition colonies.

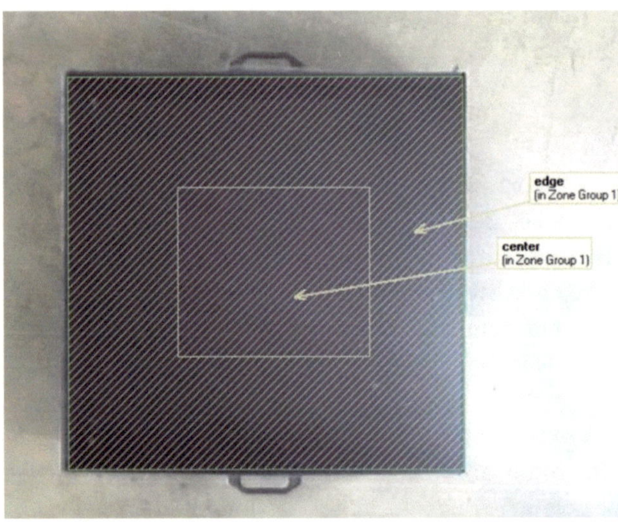

Figure 1. The edge and the center of the open field are seen.

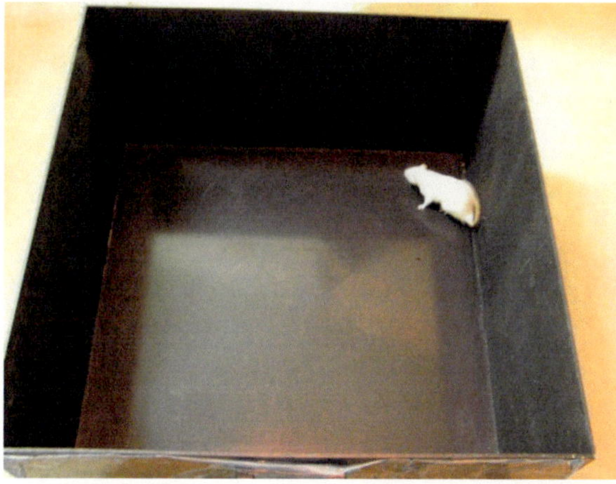

Figure 2. Rat is seen in the open field.

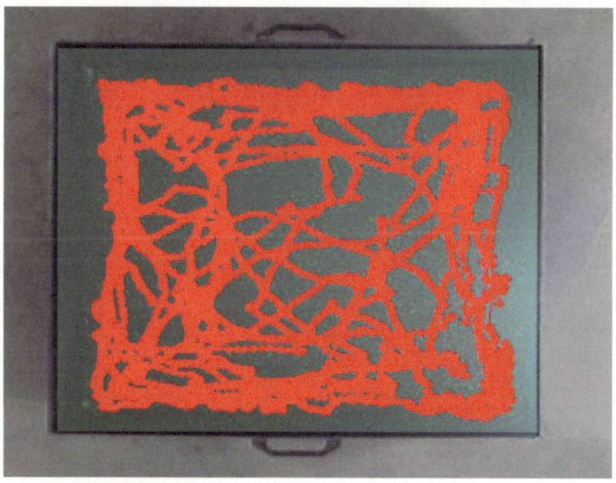

Figure 3. Total distance travelled is high. The anxiety-like behaviour is low.

2.8. Elevated plus maze

The elevated plus maze consisted of the two open and two closed 10 cm wide arms in a plus-sign configuration 55 cm off the floor. The closed arms were enclosed by 41 cm tall black Plexiglas. All arms were covered with contact paper to prevent the animals from sliding off, and all surfaces were wiped with 70% alcohol between animals. Each animal was released into one of the closed arms and allowed to move freely on the maze for a 5-min testing period that was videotaped from above the maze. Animals that fell off the maze into compartments below were placed back on the maze for the remainder of the testing period. An observer uninformed about experimental conditions scored the videotapes with the Observer Software (EthoVision XT) (Noldus Ethovision, Version 6, Netherland; Commat LTD.ŞTİ. Ankara/Turkey) for distance, duration in the open arm, frequency in the open arm, duration in the closed arms, frequency in the closed arms, mobility, and velocity. Animals were considered to have entered an arm when all four paws crossed onto the arm.

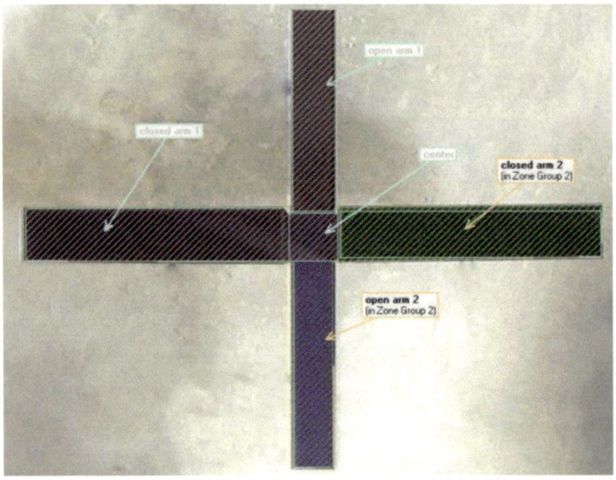

Figure 4. Open and closed arms of the elevated plus maze are seen.

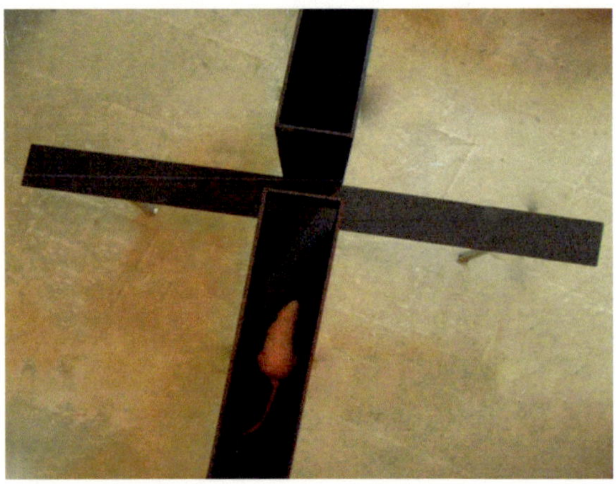

Figure 5. Rat is seen in the closed arm of the elevated plus maze.

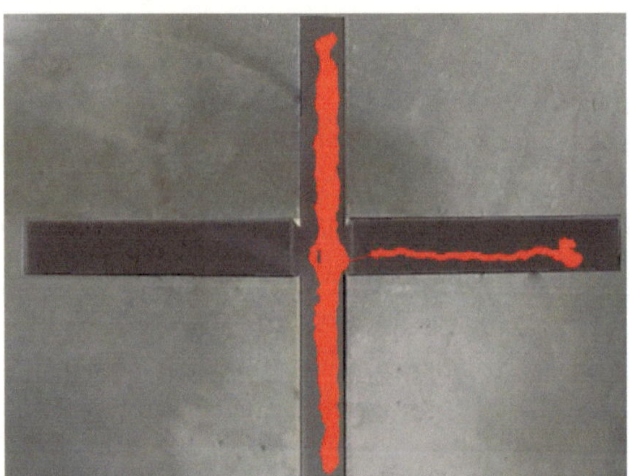

Figure 6. Time spent in open arm is high. The anxiety is low.

2.9. Morris water maze

For the spatial memory, the performance in the Morris water maze was evaluated. The experiments were carried out in a circular, galvanized steel maze (1,5 m in diameter and 60 cm in depth), which was filled with 40 cm deep water kept at 28 °C and rendered opaque by the addition of a non-toxic, water soluble dye. The maze was located in a large quiet test room, surrounded by many visual cues external to the maze (e.g. the experimenter, ceiling lights, rack, pictures, etc.), which were visible from within the pool and could be used by the rats for spatial orientation. The locations of the cues were unchanged throughout the period of testing. A video camera fixed to the ceiling over the center of the maze was used for recording and monitoring movements of the animals. There were the four equally divided quadrants in the pool. In one of the quadrants, a platform (1.0 cm below water surface, 10 cm in diameter) was submerged centrally and fixed in position which was kept constant throughout the acquisition or probe trials. The rats performed the five trials per day for the four consecutive days (20 trials). In the swimming trials each individual rat was released gently into the water at a randomly chosen quadrant except for the one that contained the hidden platform for facing an extra maze cue. The rat swam and learned how to find the hidden platform within 60 s. After reaching, the rat was allowed to stay on the platform for 15 s and was then taken back into the cage. During the inter-trial intervals, the rats were kept in a dry home cage for 60 s.

In order to assess the spatial memory, the platform was kept away from the maze for 24 hours in the final trial. Each rat was placed into the water as in the training trials and the time in seconds spent in the quadrant formerly occupied by the platform (correct quadrant) was recorded. The platform remained in the same quadrant during the entire experiment. The rats were required to find the platform using only the distal spatial cues available in the testing room. The cues were kept constant throughout the testing.

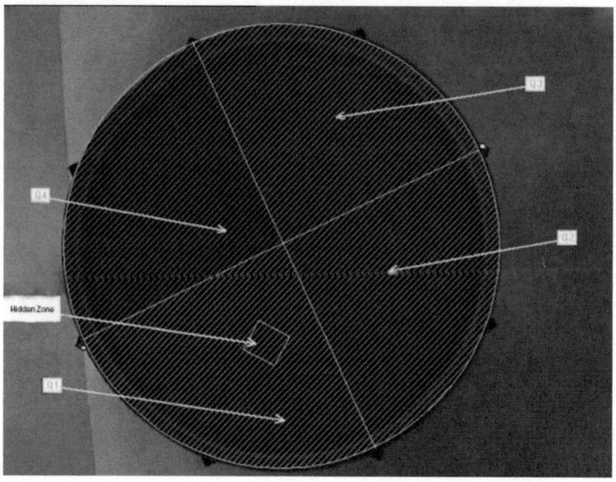

Figure 7. The quarters of the water maze and the hidden platform are seen.

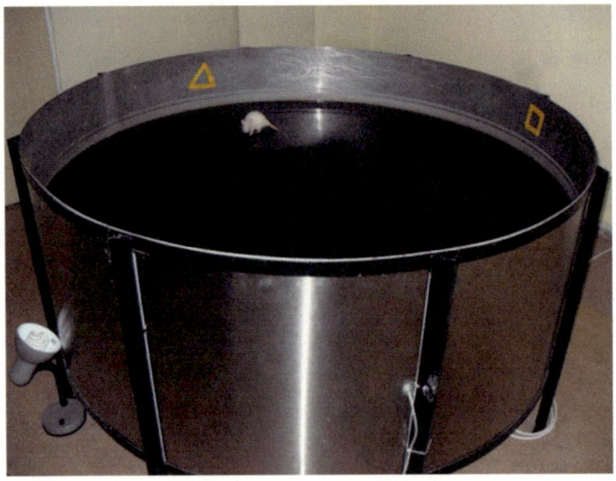

Figure 8. Rat is on the platform after it found the hidden platform.

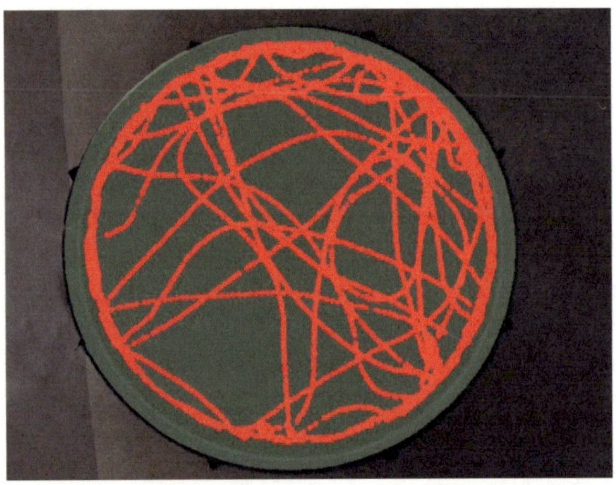

Figure 9. Total distance travelled is high. Time to find the platform is long.

2.10. Statistical analyses

Data were analyzed using SPSS (SPSS Statistical Software, SPSS Inc., Los Angeles, CA, USA, Ver. 15.0). A 2 (pinealectomy and control) X 4 (treatments: saline, diazepam, 1 μg/kg melatonin and 100 μg/kg melatonin) ANOVA analyses on data were performed with the last factor as a within subject or repeated design. Significant ANOVA results were also tested by the post test, namely the Tukey test which is assumed to be a strong test for comparison of groups that has equal variance and sample size. Values were considered statistically significant at $p \leq 0.05$. Data are presented as MEAN ± SEM after back transforming from ANOVA results.

3. Results

3.1. Anxiety measures

3.1.1. Open field measurements

3.1.1.1. Total distance travelled

An interaction effect between the group and the treatment was significant on the total distance travelled on the open field, $F(3, 36) = 6.15$, $p < 0.002$, $\eta^2 = .34$. This effect reflected the fact that in control condition subjects received 100 μg/kg melatonin (M = 699.65) and 1 μg/kg melatonin (M = 690.46) treatments travelled less distance than those received diazepam (M = 1400.04) and saline (M = 1214.95), whereas in the pinealectomy condition, the subjects received diazem (M = 643.75) travelled less distance than those received 100 μg/kg melatonin (M = 1070.22), 1 μg/kg melatonin (M = 914.38) and saline (M = 902.11) treatments.

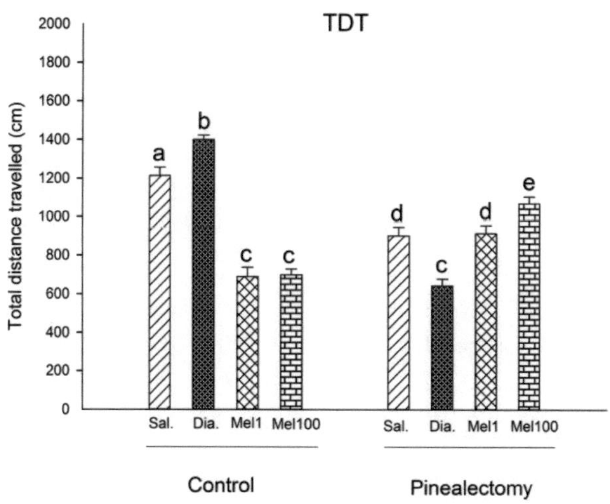

Figure 10. The total distance travelled. Right striated bar represents the saline injection and black bar represents diazepam injections, cross striated bar represents 1 μg/kg melatonin injection and bricks striated bar represents 100 μg/kg melatonin injection for both control and pinealectomy groups. Data are presented as means (± S.E.M.). Different letters indicate the statistically different groups. (Reproduced with permission from Karakas et al.; published by Elsevier, 2011a.)

3.1.1.2. Time spent at the edge of the open field (Edge duration)

An interaction effect between the group and the treatment was also significant, $F\ (3, 36) = 5.38$, $p = .004$, $\eta^2 = .31$. Indicating that in control condition subjects received diazepam spent less time than the other treatments whereas, in pinealectomy condition the subjects were not significantly different from each other.

3.1.1.3. Time spent at the center of the open field (Center duration)

The interaction effect between the group and the treatment was also significant, $F(3, 36) = 5.29$, $p < 0.004$, $\eta^2 = .31$. Indicating that in control condition subjects received diazepam spent more time than the other treatments whereas, in pinealectomy condition the subjects were not significantly different from each other.

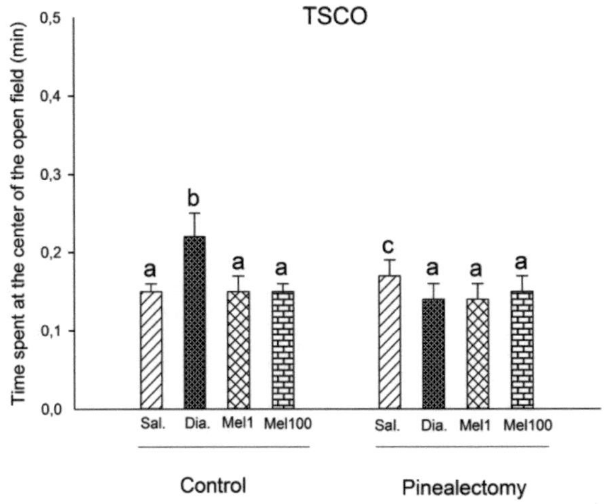

Figure 11. The time spent at the center of the open field. The bar explanations can be seen in Figure 10. (Reproduced with permission from Karakas et al.; published by Elsevier, 2011a.)

3.1.1.4. Entrance frequency to the edge of the open field (Edge frequency)

The interaction effect between the group and the treatment was significant, $F(3, 36) = 3.02$, $p < 0.04$, $\eta^2 = .20$, reflecting the fact that in control condition subjects received diazepam entered more frequently to the edge of the open field than the other treatments, whereas in pinealectomy condition the subjects who received saline treatment entered more frequently than the other treatments.

3.1.1.5. Entrance frequency to the center of the open field (Center frequency)

The interaction effect between the group and the treatment was significant, $F(3, 36) = 3.02$, $p < 0.04$, $\eta^2 = .20$, reflecting the fact that in control condition subjects received diazepam entered more frequently to the center of the open field than the other treatments, whereas in pinealectomy condition the subjects who received saline treatment entered more frequently than the other treatments.

3.1.1.6. Mobility

The main effect of the group was significant, $F\ (1, 36) = 6.89$, $p = .01$, $\eta^2 = .16$. Control group was more mobile than pinealectomy group. The main effect of the treatment was also significant, $F\ (3, 36) = 6.73$, $p = .001$, $\eta^2 = .36$. The subjects who received saline were more mobile on the open field than the other subjects with each being not significantly different from each other.

In addition, the interaction effect between the group and the treatment was significant, $F(3, 36) = 7.08$, $p < 0.001$, $\eta^2 = .37$. This reflected the fact that in control condition subjects received saline was more mobile than the other treatments, whereas in pinealectomy condition the subjects who received 100 μg/kg melatonin treatment were more mobile than the other treatments.

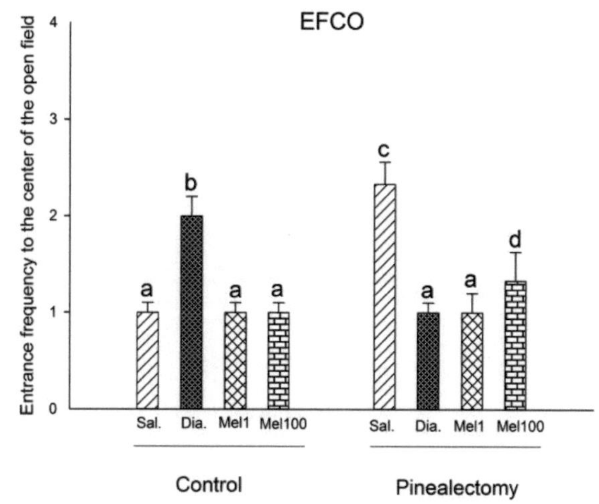

Figure 12. The entrance frequency to the center of the open field. The bar explanations can be seen in Figure 10. (Reproduced with permission from Karakas et al.; published by Elsevier, 2011a.)

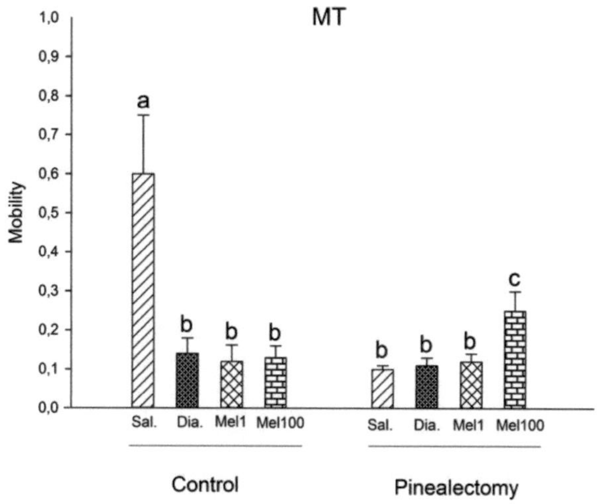

Figure 13. The mobility time . The bar explanations can be seen in Figure 10. (Reproduced with permission from Karakas et al.; published by Elsevier, 2011a.)

3.1.1.7. Velocity

The interaction effect between the group and the treatment was significant, F (3, 36) = 6.52, $p < 0.001$, $\eta^2 = .35$, indicating that in control condition subjects received saline and diazepam were faster than the other treatments, whereas in pinealectomy condition the subjects who received 100 μg/kg melatonin treatment were faster than the other treatments.

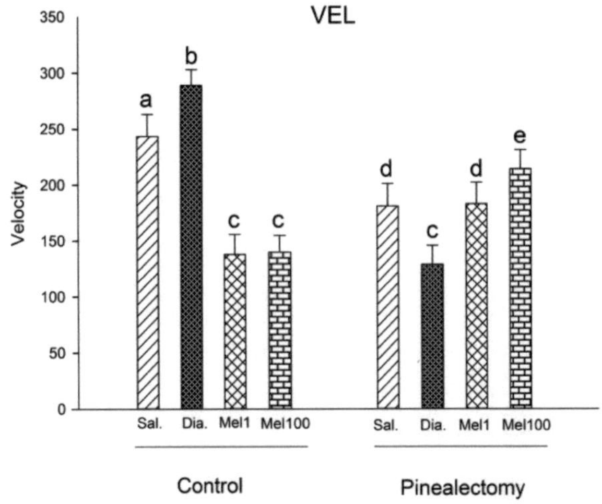

Figure 14. The velocity. The bar explanations can be seen in Figure 10. (Reproduced with permission from Karakas et al.; published by Elsevier, 2011a.)

3.1.2. Elevated plus maze measurements

3.1.2.1. Total distance travelled

The main effect of the treatment was significant, F (3, 39) = 3.06, p = .04, η^2 = .19. The groups who received diazepam travelled less distance than those who received 100 µg/kg melatonin treatments. No other differences were found to be significant.

The interaction effect between the group and the treatment was also significant on the total distance travelled on elevated plus maze, F (3, 39) = 6.52, p = 0.001, η^2 = .33. This interaction effect reflected the fact that in control condition, the subjects received diazepam travelled less distance than the other treatments, whereas in pinealectomy condition 100 µg/kg melatonin treatments travelled less distance than other treatments, whereas in the pinealectomy condition, the subjects received 100 µg/kg melatonin travelled less distance than the other treatments.

3.1.2.2. Time spent in open arms (Open arm duration)

The main effect of the treatment was significant, F (3, 39) = 6.53, p = .001, η^2 = .33. The subjects who received 100 µg/kg melatonin treatment spent more time in open arms than those who received other treatments.

An interaction effect between the group and the treatment was also significant, F (3, 39) = 6.87, $p < 0.001$, η^2 = .35. This effect indicated that in control condition subjects received 100 µg/kg melatonin treatment spent more time than those receiving the other treatments, whereas in pinealectomy condition the subjects who received saline, 100 µg/kg melatonin and diazepam treatments spent more time than those who received 1 µg/kg melatonin treatment.

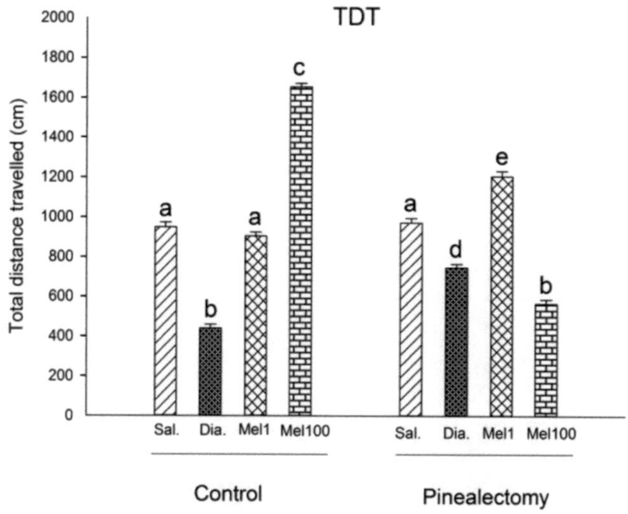

Figure 15. The total distance travelled. Right striated bar represents the saline injection and black bar represents diazepam injections, cross striated bar represents 1 μg/kg melatonin injection and bricks striated bar represents 100 μg/kg melatonin injection for both control and pinealectomy groups. Data are presented as means (± S.E.M.). Different letters indicate the statistically different groups. (Reproduced with permission from Karakas et al.; published by Elsevier, 2011a.)

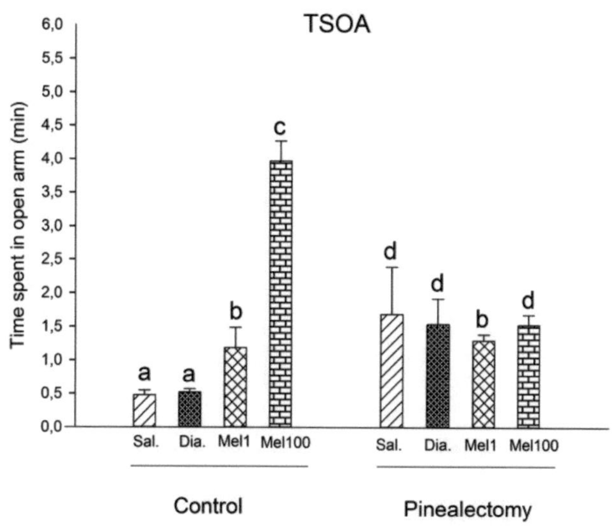

Figure 16. The time spent in open arms (TSOA). The bar explanations can be seen in Figure 15. (Reproduced with permission from Karakas et al.; published by Elsevier, 2011a.)

3.1.2.3. Time spent in closed arms (Closed arm duration)

The main effect of the treatment was significant, F (3, 39) = 6.56, p = .001, η^2 = .34. The subjects who received 100 μg/kg melatonin treatment spent less time in closed arms than those who received other treatments.

An interaction effect between the group and the treatment was also significant, F (3, 39) = 7.30, $p < 0.001$, $\eta^2 = .36$. This interaction effect reflected the fact that in control condition subjects received 100 μg/kg melatonin treatment spent less time than those receiving the other treatments, but there were no significant differences between treatment conditions in pinealectomy.

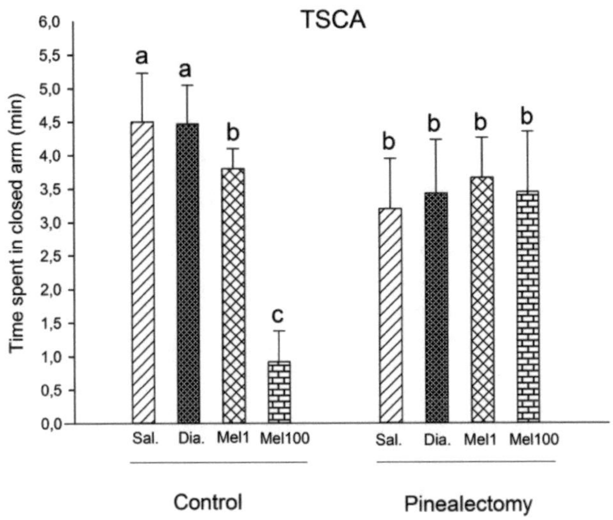

Figure 17. The time spent in closed arms (TSCA). The bar explanations can be seen in Figure 15. (Reproduced with permission from Karakas et al.; published by Elsevier, 2011a.)

3.1.2.4. Entrance frequency to open arms

The main effect of the group was significant, F (1, 39) = 14.40, $p = .001$, $\eta^2 = .27$. The subjects in the control condition entered more frequently to open arm than those in the pinealectomy.

The main effect of the treatment was also significant, F (3, 39) = 19.39, $p = .0001$, $\eta^2 = .60$. The subjects who received 100 μg/kg melatonin treatment entered more frequently to the open arm than those who received other treatments.

In addition, the interaction effect between the group and the treatment was significant, F (3, 39) = 37.65, $p = 0.0001$, $\eta^2 = .74$. This reflected the fact that in control condition subjects who received 100 μg/kg melatonin treatment entered more frequently than those who received the other treatments, whereas in pinealectomy condition the subjects who received saline, 1 μg/kg melatonin and diazepam treatments entered more frequently than those who received 100 μg/kg melatonin treatment.

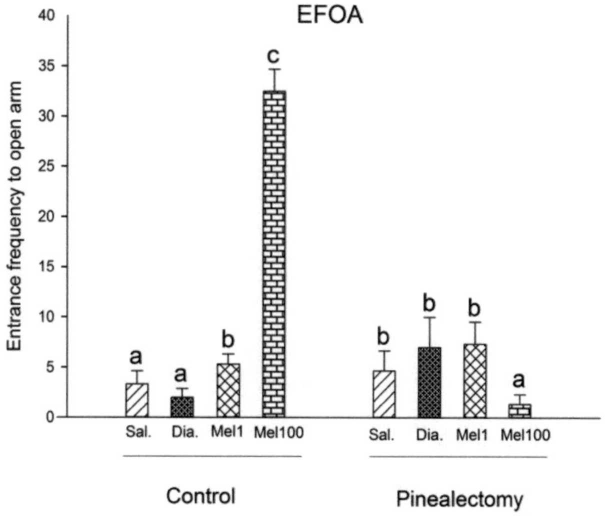

Figure 18. The entrance frequency to the open arms (EFOA). The bar explanations can be seen in Figure 15. (Reproduced with permission from Karakas et al.; published by Elsevier, 2011a.)

3.1.2.5. Entrance frequency to closed arms

No significant effects were found with regard to the total entrance to the closed arm of the elevated plus maze.

3.1.2.6. Mobility

The main effect of the group was significant, F (1, 39) = 6.95, p = .01, η^2 = .15. The subjects in the pinealectomy condition were more mobile than those in the control condition.

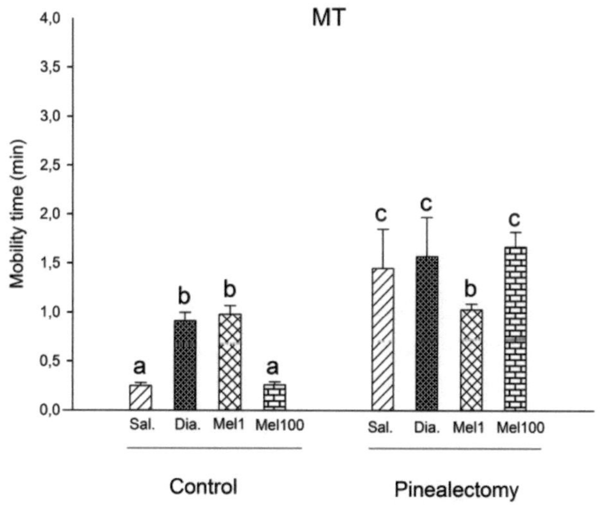

Figure 19. The mobility time (MT). The bar explanations can be seen in Figure 15. (Reproduced with permission from Karakas et al.; published by Elsevier, 2011a.)

3.1.2.7. *Velocity*

No significant effects were found with regard to the total entrance to the closed arm of the elevated plus maze.

3.1.3. *Spatial memory measures (Morris water maze measures)*

3.1.3.1. *Total distance travelled*

The interaction effect between the group and the treatment was significant on the total distance travelled on elevated plus maze, $F(3, 40) = 4.84$, $p = 0.006$, $\eta^2 = .27$. This reflected the fact that in control condition, the subjects received diazepam travelled more distance than the other treatments, whereas in pinealectomy condition subjects who reveived 100 μg/kg melatonin and the saline treatments travelled more distance than those who received 1 μg/kg melatonin and diazepam treatments.

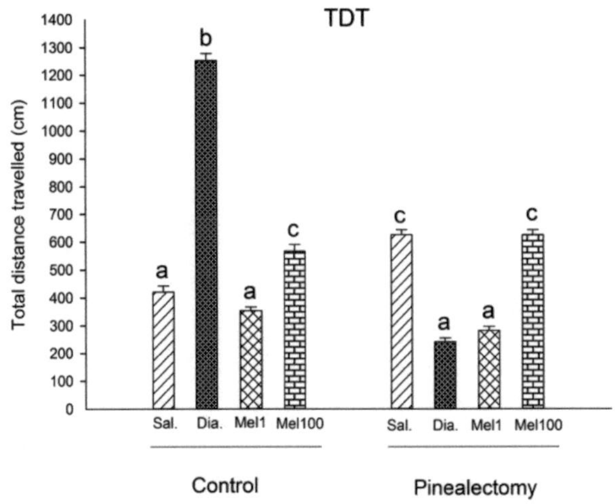

Figure 20. The total distance travelled (TDT). Right striated bar represents the saline injection and black bar represents diazepam injections, cross striated bar represents 1 μg/kg melatonin injection and bricks striated bar represents 100 μg/kg melatonin injection for both control and pinealectomy groups. Data are presented as means (± S.E.M.). Different letters indicate the statistically different groups. (Reproduced with permission from Karakas et al.; published by Elsevier, 2011a.)

3.1.3.2. *Time spent to find the platform (Latency)*

The main effect of the treatment was significant, $F\ (3, 40) = 3.02$, $p = .04$, $\eta^2 = .19$. The subjects who received diazepam treatment spent more time than those who received 1 μg/kg melatonin treatment.

In addition, the interaction effect between the group and the treatment was also significant, $F\ (3, 40) = 4.90$, $p = 0.005$, $\eta^2 = .41$. This interaction effect reflected the fact that there were no significant differences between control and pinealectomy groups in 100 μg/kg and 1 μg/kg melatonin treatments but was significant differences between these groups in saline and diazepam treatments.

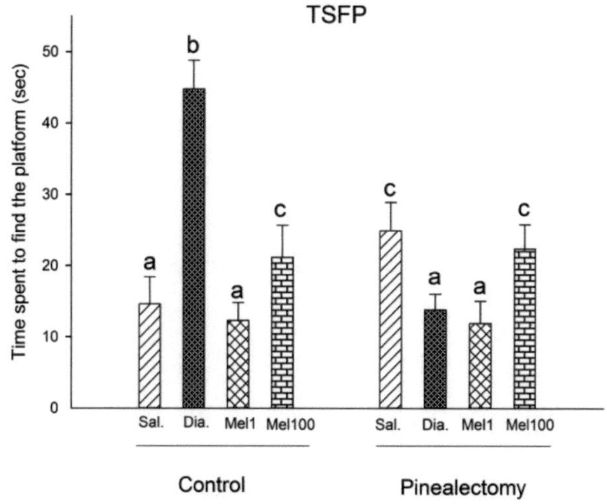

Figure 21. The time spent to find the platform (TSFP) The bar explanations can be seen in Figure 20. (Reproduced with permission from Karakas et al.; published by Elsevier, 2011a.)

3.1.3.3. Time spent in the correct quadrant

The main effect of the treatment was also significant, F (3, 40) = 4.11, p = .01, η^2 = .24. The subjects who received 1 μg/kg melatonin treatment spent less time than those who received other treatments with each being not significant from each other.

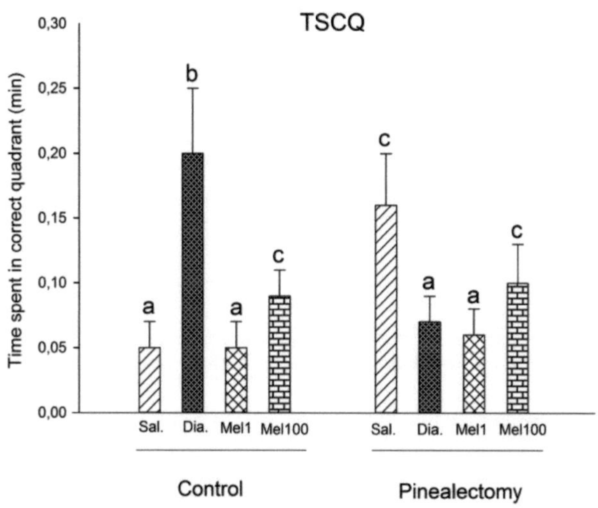

Figure 22. The time spent in the correct quadrant (TSCQ). The bar explanations can be seen in Figure 20. (Reproduced with permission from Karakas et al.; published by Elsevier, 2011a.)

In addition, the interaction effect between the group and the treatment was also significant, F (3, 40) = 9.29, p = 0.001, η^2 = .41, indicating that in control condition subjects who received diazepam treatment spent more time than those who received the other treatments, whereas in pinealectomy condition the subjects who received saline treatments spent more time than those who received other treatments.

3.1.3.4. The entrance frequency to the correct quadrant

The interaction effect between the group and the treatment was significant, $F(3, 40) = 6.72$, $p = 0.001$, $\eta^2 = .34$, indicating that in control condition subjects who received diazepam entered more frequently those who received the other treatments, whereas in pinealectomy condition the subjects who received saline treatments entered more frequently than those who received other treatments.

3.1.3.5. Mobility

No significant effects were found with regard to the mobility in the Morris water maze.

3.1.3.6. Velocity

The main effect of the group was significant, $F\ (1, 40) = 11.31$, $p = .002$, $\eta^2 = .22$. The subjects in the control condition were faster than those in the pinealectomy condition.

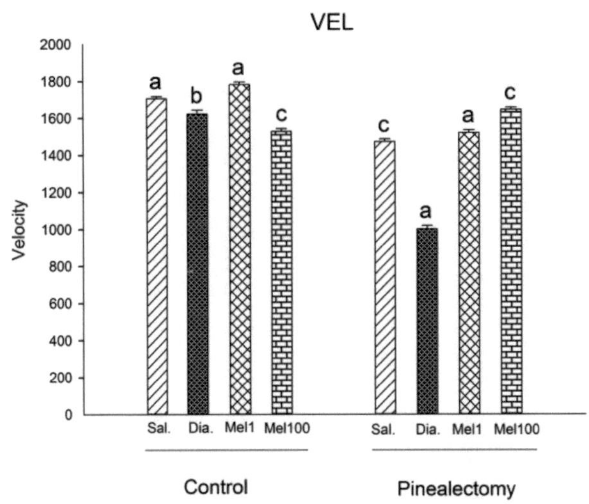

Figure 23. The velocity (VEL) are represented for the Morris water maze. The bar explanations can be seen in Figure 20. (Reproduced with permission from Karakas et al.; published by Elsevier, 2011a.)

The main effect of the treatment was also significant, $F\ (3, 40) = 4.16$, $p = .01$, $\eta^2 = .24$. The subjects who received diazepam treatment were slower than those who received other treatments.

In addition, the interaction effect between the group and the treatment was significant, $F\ (3, 40) = 4.13$, $p = 0.01$, $\eta^2 = .24$. This interaction effect reflected the fact that in control condition subjects who received 100 μg/kg melatonin treatment were slower than those who received the other treatments, whereas in pinealectomy condition, the subjects who received diazepam were slower than those who received other treatments.

3.2. Evaluation of the correct placement of the cannula

After all experiments finished, animals were decapitated and the brains were removed. We checked the placement of the cannulas histologically whether they were placed to the amygdala of the brain or not. Figure 24 represents a histological section of a brain which the cannula was placed correctly.

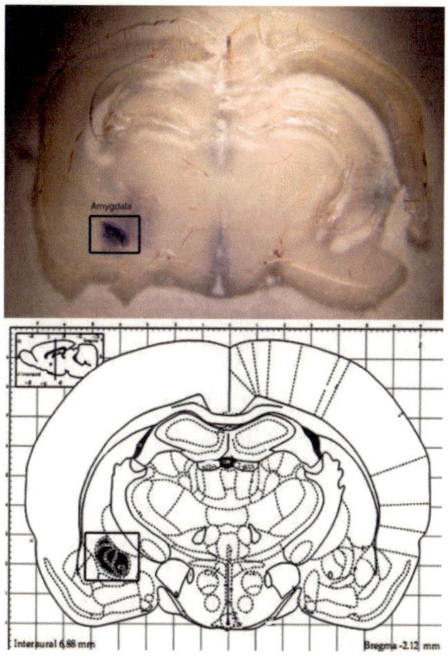

Figure 24. The figure represents the amydala region of the brain where the injections were applied. Blue colored region of the brain represents the amygdala region. (Reproduced with permission from Karakas et al.; published by Elsevier, 2011a.)

4. Discussion

The results of the present study can be described under the two main headings: anxiety-like behaviour (in open field apparatus and elevated plus maze) and spatial memory performance (in Morris water maze).

4.1. Anxiety-like behaviours

Open field test is used to measure the anxiety like behaviors in rodents (Benabid et al. 2008). The total distance traveled, the total number of entries to the center and the edge of the open field, the time spent in the center of the open field versus time spent at the edge of the open field and the mobility are frequently used parameters measured in open field test in the literature (Pyter and Nelson, 2006). In this maze, if the anxiety of the animal is high, (a) the number of the entries to the edge of the open field tends to increase, whereas that of entries to the center of the open field decrease, (b) the time passed at the edge of the open field increases, while the time passed at the center of the open field decreases, and (c) the total distance traveled, mobility and velocity in the open field decrease. The total number of the entries into the center and the edges provides a built-in control measure for general hyperactivity or sedation.

In sum, our findings were in open field that a) diazepam was more effective in reducing the anxiety since the time passed at the center of the open field was longer especially than those the 0,1 melatonin administration treatments, b) the control subjects were more mobile than the pinealectomized ones, and c) 100 μg/kg melatonin administration in contrast to other treatment conditions reduced the velocity of the animals.

Our findings reflected the fact that diazepam was more effective in reducing the anxiety. This effect was expected since the diazepam inhibits the serotonergic activity via GABAergic system. Benzodiazepines are widely used in reducing the anxiety-like behaviours. They are preferred because of their effectiveness and wide therapeutic index. They make their effect by binding their receptors which are found near the GABA receptors and by making an allosteric effect. By this way, they increase the affinity of these GABA receptors to benzodiazepines (Sinclair and Nutt, 2007). There is also possibility that amygdala also plays an important role on anxiety. The high serotonergic activity in amygdala may be one plausible explanation for this important role. This role of amygdala is supported by some research evidence that (a) a serotonin receptor agonist increased behavioral indices of anxiety without altering general activity level, and (b) a $GABA_A$ receptor agonist treatment to the medial nucleus of the amygdala inhibited escape behavior in elevated T maze.

The second finding was that there was the biggest difference in between the controls and the pinealectomies in mobility. This means that mobility measurement is more sensitive to the removal of pineal gland. It should be kept in mind that such effect was not observed in terms of other indices of the anxiety-like behaviours in this study. This finding also suggests that the amount and the rhythm of the endogeneous melatonin release in the pinealectomized animals is abolished; however, this endogeneous rhythm in the sham pinealectomized animals is intact. Therefore, the plausible effect of external high dose of melatonin administration may not become evident.

Our results, which showed that the anxiety like behaviour was not significantly affected by the pinealectomy in rats, are in good agreement with the findings of the previous studies indicating that pinealectomy alone did not have a significant effect on anxiety behavior [Kovacs et al., 1974; Juszcak et al., 1996). This suggests that the pineal gland is partially involved in the anxiety-like behaviours. The third finding was that the high dose of melatonin (100 μg/kg) administrations reduced the velocity of the animals. This effect of melatonin might be due to the direct inhibition of locomotor activity, rather than an effect on the circadian clock.

The elevated plus maze has been one of widely used tests to measure the anxiety like behaviours (Dawson and Tricklebank, 1995). In this test, the total distance traveled, the total number of entries to the closed and open arms, the time spent in closed and open arms, the mobility and the velocity are used parameters measured. In this maze, if the anxiety of the animal is high, (a) the number of the entries to closed arms increases whereas those to open arms decreases, (b) the time passed in closed arm increases whereas that passed in open arms decreases and (c) the total distance traveled, mobility and velocity decrease. The total number of the entries into all arms provides a built-in control measure for general hyperactivity or sedation.

In sum, our findings were in elevated plus maze that, a) the high dose (100 μg/kg) of melatonin increased the distance totally travelled, whereas such dose after pinealectomy decreased it, b) 100 μg/kg melatonin increased the time spent in open arms; however, after the pinealectomy, the low dose of melatonin (1 μg/kg) decreased it and c) pinealectomized animals were more mobile than control ones.

The increase in travelled distance induced by high dose of melatonin administration was reversed by the pinealectomy. This suggests that internal melatonin concentrations and rhythm may be more likely to change the effects of exogeneous melatonin administration in the anxiety like behaviors. It is well known fact that pinealectomy abolishes the rhythmic endogenous melatonin release and decreases the plasma levels of melatonin significantly (Hoffman and Reiter, 1965). Thus, after the removal of the pineal gland a high dose of melatonin could show its effect on anxiety-like behavior. The second finding in the elevated plus maze was that the high dose of melatonin increased the time spent in open arms, while, after the pinealectomy, the low dose of melatonin decreased it. In the literature, there is evidence for the interaction of melatonin with central gama aminobutyric acid (GABA) neurotransmission. Melatonin has been shown to increase the GABA levels in rat brain tissue *in vitro* (Niles et al., 1987; Coloma and Niles, 1988). When melatonin was applied *in vivo*, it increased the GABA levels in several brain regions in rats (Rosenstein and Cardinali, 1986; Xu et al., 1995). In conclusion, our findings can be attributed the fact that high dose of melatonin increased the GABA levels, which in turns reduce anxiety like behaviors. Through this mechanism, the high dose of melatonin administered subjects spent more time in open arms than the others.

The third finding in the elevated plus maze was that pinealectomy increased the mobility time in compared to controls. This finding suggests that mobility measurement is more sensitive to the removal of pineal gland. One can see that this effect was opposite of what was found in open arms. This difference may be due to the task difference between open field and elevated plus maze. Motor functions such as spontaneous activity is measured by the open field. Open field test is also used to measure the anxiety like behavior in rodents (Benabid et al., 2008). The total distance traveled, the total number of entries to the center and the edge of the open field, the time spent in the center of the open field versus time spent at the edge of the open field and the mobility are frequently used parameters measured in open field test in the literature (Pyter and Nelson, 2006). In this maze, if the anxiety of the animal is high, the number of the entries to the edge of the open field is increasing and the total distance traveled is decreasing. The total number of the entries into the center and the edges provides a built-in control measure for general hyperactivity or sedation. On the other hand, the elevated plus maze has been one of popular or widely used test to measure the anxiety like behaviors (Dawson and Tricklebank, 1995). In this maze, if the anxiety of the animal is high, the number of the entries to closed arms is increasing and the total distance traveled is decreasing. The total number of the entries into all arms provides a built-in control measure for general hyperactivity or sedation. Regarding elevated plus maze and open field tests, the present study represent a difference in mobility, which needs a further investigation. Our findings also suggest that the elevated plus maze condition provides melatonin specific outcomes more than the open field condition.

4.2. Spatial memory performance

The Morris water maze has been one of widely used tests to measure the spatial memory performance. In this maze, the time passed to find the platform, total distance travelled, the frequency of the entrance to the correct quadrant, the time passed in correct quadrant, mobility and velocity parameters are measured (Morris, 1984).

In this study,(a) diazepam administration increased the total distance travelled more than the others in the control condition whereas, in the pinealectomy condition the high dose of melatonin and saline groups travelled more distance than the others,(b) in the pinealectomy condition, the subjects with the high dose of melatonin also travelled more distance than those with the low dose of melatonin and diazepam, (c) the subjects who received 1 μg/kg melatonin spent less time than those who received other treatments, and (d) in the control condition, the subjects with the high dose of melatonin treatment were slower than those who received the other treatments. Longer distance travelled and less time spent in the correct quadrant indicates less spatial learning in this maze. It should be especially noted that the high doses of melatonin decreased some behavioral indices of spatial memory. In line with this finding, other studies have consistently shown that amygdala damage through various implementations leads to the impairment of learning an association between an auditory cue and food reward (Sutherland and Mc Donalds, 1990), of performance on conditioned place preference task (McIntyre et al., 1998), and working memory (Addy et al., 2003). It is a well known fact that melatonin readily passes all cell membranes, including the blood-brain barrier (Reiter et al., 1993). Melatonin binding sites exist in various brain structures such as the hippocampus and prefrontal cortex are considered to involve in memory function (Brzezinski, 1997; Ekmekçioğlu, 2006; Mazzuchelli et al., 1996; Savaskan et al., 2001; 2005). Moreover, considering that melatonin is a potent sleep inducing enhanced consolidation of hippocampus-dependent memories (Jern et al., 1991; Rasch et al., 2007), it is possible that 'sleep-like' melatonin effects on consolidation in the aftermath of encoding added to its effects on encoding. Despite this evidence, exact mechanism of melatonin concerning cognitive performance is still not known and there are some plausible explanations.

One explanation deals with its pathway. Melatonin could have direct or indirect effect on memory. Some studies have provided evidence for its direct effect. For instance, a research has suggested that melatonin could be involved in structural remodeling of synaptic connections during memory and learning processes (Baydas et al., 2002). Other research has also suggested that melatonin may influence memory formation in the hippocampus (El Sherif et al., 2003). In addition to its direct action, indirectly, melatonin may act as an antioxidant to reduce oxidative damage to the synapses in hippocampus and therefore improves learning and memory deficits. Tuzcu and Baydas (2006) have found evidence indicating that melatonin significantly ameliorated the cognitive impairment, reduced lipid per oxidation, and increased glutathione levels in diabetic rats. In conclusion, the effect of melatonin on learning performance could be in both ways. Even though the present study was not aimed to directly test this explanation, its results suggest that melatonin injection seems to have direct effect on spatial memory that has been related to limbic system of rat brain. Melatonin may also have an indirect effect on learning performance via some neurotransmitter such as gama amino butyric acid (GABA). An increase in melatonin level via injection may also affect the GABA, an inhibitory neurotransmitter, which in turn may decrease the neural transmission in the limbic system. Through this way, melatonin microinjection to amygdala may show its impairing effect on learning and memory processes. In addition to the regulatory role of amygdala in anxiety, amygdala is of great importance in regulating memory and learning functions. The removal of the temporal lobe in animals leads to an impairment in memory in a way that the subjects experience difficulties in learning new material after the removal of amygdala. Also, damage to amygdala leads to an impairment of learning an association between an auditory cue and food reward. In addition, the muscarinic receptor antagonist administration to amygdala impaired performance on conditioned place preference task (McIntyre et al., 1998). Moreover, the nicotinic receptor antagonist administrations impair working memory (Addy et al., 2003). The results of our study indicate that the administration of melatonin to amygdala with the abolishment of melatonin hormone via pinealectomy produced different effects on anxiety-like and learning behaviors.

In addition, melatonin may also show its effects through its reciprocal relationship with some parts of rat brain such as suprachiasmatic nucleus (SCN). While SCN is generating and controlling the circadian rhythm of melatonin, melatonin hormone is also acting on SCN as a negative feedback agent in order to control the activity of the SCN. It is well known fact that the release of the melatonin hormone in rats shows a circadian pattern which is high throughout the darkness (Klein, 1974). However, in pinealectomy the blood melatonin levels drop significantly and the rhythm of melatonin is abolished (Chapman, 1970).

The other explanation for the effects of melatonin on learning performance is related with the circadian effects of melatonin. Several studies have demonstrated the regulatory roles of melatonin in circadian rhythms (Brzezinski, 1997; Borjigin et al., 1999; Arendt, 2000). For instance, our recent experiment has shown that daily injections of melatonin can entrain the activity rhythms of the pinealectomized Mongolian gerbils (*Meriones unguiculatus*) (unpublished data). This effect of melatonin might be due to the direct inhibition of locomotor activity, rather than an effect on the circadian clock.

It should be kept in mind that we implemented microinjections in the afternoon when the melatonin receptors are re-sensitive to the melatonin hormone. According to the internal coincidence hypothesis, melatonin exerts an effect only when its circadian secretion is coincident with target tissue sensitivity. This hypothesis supposes that the time of presence of melatonin is important (Stetson and Tay, 1983; Hong and Stetson, 1987). In line with this explanation, we found in our another study that pinealectomy and only admistration of melatonin via timed injections caused impairment of the learning performance of the rats (Karakas et al., 2011b).

4.3. Conclusion

In conclusion, the results of the present experiment have indicated that the data coming from the elevated plus maze and the open field are consistent to each other. However, our results have suggested that elevated plus maze measurements were more sensitive to the melatonin microinjections to amygdala than open field measurements, since the differences were more evident in this maze. This suggests that pinealectomy treatment interacts with anxiety provoking test situations. In open field, it was assumed that the anxiety level experience by animals may be greater in elevated plus maze than open field. In open field the mobility was smaller in pinealectomized rats than controls since the anxiety level may be low compared to the elevated plus maze. This explanation requires further experimental research that illuminates differential effects of pinealectomy on testing conditions.

Taken together, these results are unique contribution to the field of anxiety like behavior and spatial learning in the literature. Further research should take multiple measures of anxiety and learning in the given consideration that melatonin injection produce different outcomes in the investigated parameters in open field, elevated plus maze and Morris water maze.

Author details

Alper Karakas
Department of Biology, Faculty of Arts and Sciences,
Abant Izzet Baysal University,Bolu, Turkey

Hamit Coskun
Department of Psychology, Faculty of Arts and Sciences, Abant Izzet Baysal University, Bolu, Turkey

5. References

Abrams, JK., Johnson, PL., Shekhar, A. & Lowry, CA. (2004a) Anxiogenic drugs act selectively ontopographically distinct midbrain, pontine, and medullary serotonergic neurons. *Eur Neuropsychopharm* 14, Supplement 3: S124

Abrams, JK., Johnson, PL., Shekhar, A. & Lowry, CA. (2004b) Anxiogenic drugs act selectively on topographically distinct midbrain, pontine, and medullary serotonergic neurons. *Eur Neuropsychopharm* 14, Supplement 1: S21

Addy, NA., Nakijama, A. & Levin, ED., (2003) Nicotinic mechanisms of memory: effects of acute local DH beta E andMLAinfusions in the basolateral amygdale. *Cognit Brain Res* 16, (1): 51-57

Almonte,AG., Hamill, CE., Chhatwal, JP., Wingo, TS., Barber, JA., (2007) Learning and memory deficits in mice lacking protease activated receptor-1. *Neurobiol Learn Mem* 88, *3, 295-304*

Appenrodt, E. & Schwarzberg, H. (1999) Septal vasopressin modulates motility and passive avoidance in pinealectomized rats. *Physiol Behav* 66, 757–61.

Appenrodt, E. & Schwarzberg, H. (2000) Central vasopressin administration failed to influence anxiety behavior after pinealectomy in rats. *Physiol Behav* 68, 735–9.

Appenrodt, E. & Schwarzberg, H. (2003) Pinealectomy blocks modulation of active avoidance by central vasopressin application in rats. *Peptides 24,* 129-136.

Appenrodt, E, Juszczak, M. & Schwarzberg, H. (2002) Septal vasopressininduced preservation of social recognition in rats was abolished by pinealectomy. *Behav Brain Res 134,* 67–73.

Arendt, J. (1988) Melatonin. *Clin Endocrinology* 29, 205-29

Arendt, J. (1995) *Melatonin and the mammalian pineal gland*. Chapman and Hall, London, UK.

Arendt, J. (2000) Melatonin, circadian rhythms and sleep. *New England J Med* 343, 1114-1116.

Argyriou, A., Prast, H. & Philippu, A. (1998) Melatonin facilitates short-term memory. *Eur J Pharmacol 349,* 159-162.

Baydas, G., Nedzvetsky, VS., Nerush, PA., Kırıchenko, SV., Demchenko, HM., et al.(2002) A novel role for melatonin: regulation of the expression of cell adhesion molecules in the hippocampus, cortex and cerebellum. *Neurosci Lett* 326, 109–112.

Benabid, N., Mesfıoui, A. & Ouichou, A. (2008). Effects of photoperiod regimen on emotional behaviour in two tests for anxiolytic activity in Wistar rat. *Brain Res Bull* 75, 53-59

Binkley, S. (1988) The pineal: endocrine and nonendocrine function. Prentice Hall, New Jersey, Usa

Blackshear, A., Yamamoto, M., Anderson, B.J., Holmes, P.V., Lundström, L.,et al., (2007) Intracerebroventricular administration of galanin or galanin receptor subtype 1 agonist M617 induces c-Fos activation in central amygdala and dorsomedial hypothalamus. *Peptides* 28, *5, 1120-1124*

Borjigin, J., Li, X. & Snyder, S H. (1999) The pineal gland and melatonin: molecular and pharmacologic regulation. *Annu Rev Pharmacol* 39, 53-65.

Brzezinski, A. (1997) Melatonin in humans. *New Engl J Med* 336,186-195.

Cao, X J., Wang, M., Chen, W H., Zhu, D M., She, J Q., et al., (2009) Effects of chronic administration of melatonin on spatial learning ability and long-term potentiation in lead-exposed and control Rats. *Biomed Environ Sci* 22, 70-75.

Cardinalli, DP., Vacas, MI. & Boyer, E E. (1979) Specific binding of melatonin in bovine brain. *Endocrinology* 105, 437-441.

Chapmann, D I. (1970) Seasonal changes in the gonads and accessory glands of male mammals. *Mammal Rev* 1, 231–248.

Coloma, FM. & Niles, LP. (1988) Melatonin enhancement of [3H]-gamma-aminobutyric acid and [3H] muscimol binding in rat brain. *Biochem Pharmacol* 37, 1271-1274.

Cornélio, A.M. & Luiz Nunes-de-Souza, R. (2007) Anxiogenic-like effects of mCPP microinfusions into the amygdala (but not dorsal or ventral hippocampus) in mice exposed to elevated plus-maze. *Behav Brain Res* 178, 1, 12, 82-89

Dawson, GR. & Tricklebank MD. (1995) Use of the elevated plus maze in the search for novel anxiolytic agents. *Trends Pharmacol Sci* 16 (2), pp. 33–36.

Ekmekcioglu, C. (2006) Melatonin receptors in humans: biological role and clinical revelance. *Biomed Pharmacother* 60, 97-108.

El-Sherif, Y, Tesoriero, J, Hogan, M V. & Wieraszko, A. (2003) Melatonin regulates neuronal plasticity in the hippocampus. *J Neurosci Res* 72, 454–460.

Gilman, S. & Newman, SW. (1992) *Manter and Gatz's Essentials of clinical neuroanatomy and neurophysiology*. 8. Edition Davis company Philadelphia

Golombek, DA., Pevet, P. & Cardinalli, DP. (1996) Melatonin effects on behavior: possible mediation by the central GABAergic system. *Neurosci Biobehav Rev* 20, 403-412.

Hale, M.W., Bouwknecht, J.A., Spiga, F., Shekhar, A. & Lowry, C.A. (2006) Exposure to high- and low-light conditions in an open-field test of anxiety increases c-Fos expression in specific subdivisions of the rat basolateral amygdaloid complex. *Brain Res Bull* 71, 1-3, 174-182

Herdade, KC., Strauss, CV. & Zangrossi, JH. (2006) Effects of medial amygdala inactivation on a panic related behaviour. *Behav Brain Res* 25, 172 (2) 316-23

Hoffmann, K. (1974) Testicular involution in short photoperiods inhibited by melatonin. *Naturwissenschaften* 61,364-365

Hoffman, R A. & Reiter R J. (1965) Rapid pinealectomy in hamsters and other small rodents. *Anat Record* 24, 83–89

Hong, S M. & Stetson., M H. (1987) Detailed diurnal rhythm of sensitivity to melatonin injections in Turkish hamsters. *Mesocricetus brandti. J Pineal Res* 4: 69-78.

Jern, C., Manhem, K., Eriksson, E., Tengborn, L., Risberg, B., et al. (1991) Hemostatic responses to mental stress during the menstrual cycle. *Thromb Haemostasis* 66: 614-618.

Juszcak, M., Drobnik, J., Guzek, JW. & Schwarzberg, H. (1996) Effect of pinealectomy and melatonin on vasopressin-potentiated passive avoidance in rats. *J Physiol Pharmacol* 47: 621–7.

Karakaş, A., Coşkun, H., Kaya, A., Kucuk, A. & Gunduz, B. (2011a) The Effects Of the intraamygdalar melatonin injections on the anxiety like behaviour and the spatial memory performance in male wistar rats. *Behav Brain Res* 222, 141-150,

Karakaş, A., Coşkun, H. & Kaya, A. (2011b) The effects of pinealectomy, melatonin injections and implants on the spatial memory performance of male Wistar rats. *Biol Rhythm Res* 42, (6) 457-472

Klein DC. (1974) Circadian rhythms in indole methabolism in the rat pineal gland, in *the Neurosciences*; Third study program. MIT press, Cambridge, Massachusetts, pp. 509-16

Klein, DC. 1993 The mammalian melatonin rhythm generating system. In: Watterberg L (ed). *Light and biological rhythms in man,* Pergamon Pres, New York, pp. 55-70.

Kovács, GL., Gajari, I., Telegdy, G. & Lissak, K. (1974) Effects of melatonin and pinealectomy on avoidance and exploratory activity in the rat. *Physiol Behav* 13, 349–55.

Krause, D N. & Dubocovich, M L. (1990) Regulatory sites in the melatonin system of mammals. *Trends Neurosci* 13, 464-470.

Lecourtier, L., Saboureau, M., Kelly, CD., Pevet, P. & Kelly, PH. (2005) Impaired cognitive performance in rats after complete epithalamus lesions, but not after pinealectomy alone. *Behav Brain Res* 161, 276–285.

Lerner, AB., Case, JD., Takahashi, Y., Lee, TH. & Mori, W. (1958) Isolation of melatonin, pineal factor that lightens melanocytes. *J Am Chem Soc* 80, 2587

Loiseau, F., Bihan, CL., Hamon, M. & Thiebot, MH. (2006) Effects of melatonin and agomelatine in anxiety-related procedures in rats: Interaction with diazepam. *Eur Neuropsychopharm* 16, 417-428.

Martinez, LA., Klann, E. & Tejada-Simon, MV. (2007) Translocation and activation of Rac in the hippocampus during associative contextual fear learning. *Neurobiol Learn Mem* 88, *1, 104-113*

Martini, L. (1971) Behavioral effects of pineal principles. In: Wolsten-holme, G. E. W., Knight, J. (Eds), *The pineal Gland.* Livingstone, Edinburgh pp. 368-372.

Masana, M I. & Dubocovich, M L. 2001Melatonin receptor signaling: finding the path through the dark. *Science STKE* pe39.

Mazzucchelli, C., Pannacci, M., Nonno, R., Lucini, V., Franchini, F., et al. (1996) The melatonin receptor in the human brain: cloning experiments and distribution studies. *Brain Res, Mol Brain Res* 39, 117-126.

McIntyre, CK., Ragozzino, ME. & Gold, PE. (1998) Intra-amygdala infusions of scopolamine impair performance on a conditioned place preference task but not a spatial radial maze task. *Behav Brain Res* 95, (2) 219-226

Morris, R. (1984) Developments of a water-maze procedure for studying spatial learning in the rat. *J Neurosci Methods* 11,47-60

Naranjo-Rodriguez, EB., Ortiz Orsornio, A., Hernandez-Avitia, E., Mendoza-Fernandez, V. & Escobar, A. (2000). Anxiolytic-like actions of melatonin, 5-methoxytryptophan, 5-hydroxytryptophol and benzodiazepines on a conflict procedure. *Prog Neuropsychopharmacol Biol Psychiatry* 24, 117–129.

Niles, LP., Pickering, DS. & Arciszewski MA. (1987) Effects of chronic melatonin administration on GABA and diazepam binding in rat brain. *J Neural Transm* 70,117-124.

Panke, ES., Rollag, MD. & Reiter, RJ. (1979) Pineal melatonin concentrations in the Syrian hamster. *Endocrinology* 104,197-197

Papp, M., Litwa, E., Gruca, P. & Mocaer, E. (2006) Anxiolytic-like activity of agomelatine and melatonin in three animal models of anxiety. *Behav Pharmacol* 17, 9-18.

Poeggeler, B., Saarela, S., Reiter, RJ., Tan, DX., Chen, LD., et al., (1994) Melatonin, a highly potent endogeneous radical scavenger and electron donor, new aspects of the antioxidant chemistry of this indole accessed in vitro. *Neurobiol NO OH* 738, 419-420.

Pyter, LM. & Nelson, RJ.(2006) Enduring effects of photoperiod on affective behaviors in Siberian Hamsters (Phodopus sungorus). *Behav Neurosci* 120, (1) 125-134.

Quay, WB. (1974) Pineal chemistry in cellular and physiological mechanisms. Charles C. Thomas, IL, USA

Rasch, B., Buchel, C., Gais, S. & Born, J. (2007) Odor cues during slowwave sleep prompt declarative memory consolidation. *Science* 315, 1426-1429.

Refinetti, R., Kaufman, CM. & Menaker, M. (1994) Complete suprachiasmatic lesions eliminate circadian rhythmicity of body temperature and locomotor activity in golden hamsters. J Comp Physiol A, 175, 223–232.

Reiter, RJ., Poeggeler, B., Tan, DX., Chen, LD., Manchester, LC., et al. (1993) Antioxidant capacity of melatonin: a novel action not requiring a receptor. *Neuroendocrinol Lett* 15, 103-116.

Reppert, SM. (1997) Melatonin receptors: molecular biology of a new family of G protein-coupled receptors. *J Biol Rhythm* 12,528-531

Rosenstein, RE. & Cardinali, DP. (1986) Melatonin increases in vivo Gaba accumulation in rat hypothalamus, cerebellum, cerebral cortex and pineal gland. *Brain Res* 398, 403-406

Savaskan, E., Olivieri, G., Brydon, L., Jockers, R., Krauchi, K., et al.(2001) Cerebrovascular melatonin MT1-receptor alterations in patients with Alzheimer's disease. *Neurosci Lett* 308, 9-12.

Savaskan, E., Ayoub, M A., Ravid, R., Angeloni, D., Franchini, F., et al. (2005) Reduced hippocampal MT2 melatonin receptor expression in Alzheimer's disease. *J Pineal Res* 38,10-16.

Sinclair, L. & Nutt, D. (2007) Anxiolytics. *Psychiatry* 6, 7, 284-288

Stankov, B., Fraschini, F. & Reiter, RJ. (1991) Melatonin binding sites in the central nervous system. *BrainResRev* 16,245-256.

Steinlechner, S. (1996) Melatonin as a chronobiotic: PROS and CONS. *Acta Neurobiol Exp* 56, 363-372

Stetson, M N. & Tay, D E. (1983) Time course of sensitivity of golden hamsters to melatonin injections throughout the day. *Biol Reprod* 29, 432-38.

Sugden, D. (1991) Adrenergic mechanisms regulating pineal melatonin synthesis. Adv Pineal Res 5:33-8

Sutherland, RJ. & Mc Donalds, RJ. (2006) Hippocampus, amygdale and memory deficits. *Behav Brain Res* 1990, 34, 57-79

Tuzcu, M. & Baydas, G. (2006) Effect of melatonin and vitamin E on diabetes-induced learning and memory impairment in rats. *Eur J Pharmacol* 537, 106-110.

Vanecek, J. (1999) Inhibitory effect of melatonin on GnRH induced LH release. *Rev Reprod* 4, 67-72.

Weaver, DR., Rivkees, SA. & Reppert, SM. (1989) Localization and characterization of melatonin receptors in rodent brain by in vitro aotoradiography. *J Neurosci* 9, 2581-2590.

Wirz-Justice, A. (2001) Treatment tools in chronobiology. *Rev Med Interne* 22 suppl 1,37-38.

Xu, F., Li, JC., Ma, KC. & Wang, M. (1995) Effects of melatonin on hypothalamic gamma-aminobutyric acid, aspartic acid, glutamicacid, beta-endorphin and serotonin levels in male mice. *Biol Signals* 4, 225-231

Section 2

Neuropeptides in Social Behaviors and Diseases

Chapter 3

Behavioral Roles of Oxytocin and Vasopressin

Benjamin C. Nephew

Additional information is available at the end of the chapter

http://dx.doi.org/10.5772/50422

1. Introduction

Arginine Vasopressin (AVP) and oxytocin (OXT) are peptide hormones found in most mammals that have vital physiological and behavioral actions. The major sites of AVP production are the paraventricular (PVN) and supraoptic (SON) nuclei in the hypothalamus, although AVP and its receptors are found in numerous brain nuclei and peripheral tissues. AVP's physiological roles, which are mediated through both peripheral and central mechanisms, include regulating fluid homeostasis and blood pressure. It is also an important component of the endocrine stress response through its actions in the posterior pituitary gland, where it is a secretagogue of ACTH, stimulating the release of corticosteroid stress hormones and catecholamines from the adrenal glands. The three receptor subtypes for AVP are V1a, V1b, and V2. V2 receptors mediate the fluid regulating actions of AVP in the periphery, where the behavioral and central endocrine functions of AVP are mediated by the V1a and V1b receptors in the brain. These receptors are also involved in the central control of cardiovascular activity.

Oxytocin's major physiological roles are to facilitate uterine contractions during birth through a positive feedback mechanism during the second and third stages of labor, and to mediate milk letdown. In lactating mammalian mothers, OXT initiates milk letdown in the mammary glands, and the release of OXT is stimulated by suckling. OXT has one known receptor which has several alleles. The focus of the present chapter will be on the social behavior functions of both AVP and OXT. While some of these actions are mediated the PVN and SON, several other behaviorally active brain regions will also be discussed.

The behavioral roles of oxytocin and vasopressin have been studied and characterized in several animal species over the past few decades, and these findings have recently stimulated related work in humans. While the specific direction of the effects often vary between species, the general behavioral functions of AVP and OXT, as well as several related ancestral peptides, are conserved across taxa. The study of the diversity of these systems in birds [1] and fish [2] has been particularly useful in identifying the mechanisms of the effects of these peptides on behavior. Although the behavioral roles of OXT and AVP are good examples of effective translation from animal models to clinical study for some topics, such as autism, there is still a need for increased communication and collaboration on many relevant issues, especially gender differences and stress related mood disorders. Both animal and human studies on depression and anxiety indicate that these neuropeptides have gender specific roles, and administering treatments developed in male animals and humans to females may be ineffective or have adverse consequences. The objectives of this review chapter are to present an updated summary of the gender specific behavioral roles of OXT and AVP in both animals and humans and stimulate translationally relevant gender specific studies on these hormones. The need for more female specific studies in this area is great, and this need will be underscored throughout the chapter. Behavioral topics covered include affiliation, aggression, parental behavior, depression/anxiety, and memory. Clinical topics discussed include depression, anxiety, addiction, and autism. Due to the broad scope of these objectives, this review chapter will highlight selected research and review papers on each topic, but will not be comprehensive.

2. Oxytocin in male animals

2.1. OXT and male animal affiliation

While most studies of both AVP and OXT conclude that OXT is a more important mediator of affiliative behavior in females than males, there is considerable evidence that OXT may serve important social behavior functions in males as well. The most convincing evidence for the role of OXT in affiliative behavior in animals is pair bonding in prairie voles (*Microtus ochrogaster*). These voles are relatively unique in their monogamous social structure, which is mediated by OXT and AVP activity in the brain. Central OXT infusions facilitate prairie vole pair bonding [3], which has been linked to gender specific developmental effects in male voles [4]. The distribution of OXT receptors in the brain mediates divergent social strategies in monogamous and polygamous vole species [5]. Studies of social recognition and memory in male mice, processes important for the establishment of affiliative behavior, conclude that OXT actions on social behavior are mediated by changes in recognition and social memory [6, 7]. In male rats, OXT facilitates sexual behavior through actions in the PVN [8]. In pair bonded tamarin monkeys, peripheral OXT levels vary with levels of affiliation and sexual behavior in both genders [9]. Specifically, OXT levels in male tamarins were correlated strongly with sexual behavior. In fish it has been postulated that isotocin (the teleostean homologue of OXT) is involved in courtship displays and territorial defense [10], and many of the social behavior effects of OXT are conserved across taxa [11].

2.2. OXT and male animal aggression

The recent data from stickleback fish suggest that the affiliative actions of OXT in vertebrates are associated with aggression [10]. OXT levels are highest in male sticklebacks that aggressively defend eggs and in subordinate males that fight to change their social status. Disruption of the OXT gene in male mice decreases aggression [12], yet OXT knockout mice display elevated aggression which is postulated to be the result of decreased fearfulness [13]. One potential explanation for this inconsistency is indirect effects through AVP due to the neuroanatomical and biochemical similarities between the two neuropeptide systems. The increased aggression in OXT knockout mice may be mediated by a compensatory increase in AVP in these males.

2.3. OXT and animal paternal behavior

In polygamous male meadow voles (*Microtus pennsylvanicus*), paternal experience is associated with increases in OXT receptor binding in the accessory olfactory nucleus, bed nucleus of the stria terminalis, lateral septum, and lateral amygdala [14]. It was concluded that central OXT infusion increased the tolerance of the offspring by the father. Combined treatment with both an OXT antagonist and an AVP antagonist decrease male parental behavior in reproductively naïve male prairie voles, where treatments with only one antagonist did not affect the expression of alloparenting [15]. It appears that male prairie vole paternal behavior may rely on the neural effects of both peptides. Mandarin voles (*Lasiopodomys mandarinus),* which are biparental and express parental behavior towards foster pups, increase central OXT expression following the development of male alloparental behavior. This increased expression may be mediated by elevated estrogen receptor alpha [16]. In support of this association between OXT and mammalian paternal expression, a recent primate study reported that icv OXT increased the transfer of food from fathers to their offspring [17]. Similar effects of OXT in male primates are supported by clinical data which will be discussed later in this review.

2.4. OXT and male animal models of depression and anxiety

Peripheral OXT has antidepressant effects in both young and old rats, and the effects in older rats are associated with enhanced memory [18, 19]. In the mouse tail suspension test, both systemic and central OXT decrease immobility time, which indicates that OXT decreased helplessness [20]. In contrast to these results, intracerebroventricular (icv) OXT did not affect behavior in the forced swim test of depressive like behavior in male rats selected for high or low anxiety, although it did have an anxiolytic effect [21]. Furthermore, isolated prairie vole males exhibit both anhedonia and increased plasma OXT following a resident intruder test of aggression [22]. As has been hypothesized for OXT elevation following maternal aggression, this increase could be due to the stress of the interaction, and may not be a causal factor for anhedonia. It is possible that anhedonia targeting tests of depressive behavior, such as saccharin preference or a naturally occurring reward mediated behavior (sexual behavior, maternal behavior), would reveal consistent anti-depressive actions of OXT.

2.5. OXT and male animal learning and memory

Most of the research on OXT and learning and memory has been limited to male models [23]. OXT mediates social recognition in several species [24], and male OXT knockout mice exhibit social amnesia [6], while other forms of memory are not affected. This effect on social recognition is reversed by OXT treatment [7] and is mediated by the transmembrane protein CD38 [25]. A single dose of OXT can specifically impair memory retention [26], and further study indicates that exogenous OXT inhibits cholinergic mechanisms that are necessary for memory retention [27]. Another mechanism implicated in the amnesiac effects of OXT is glucocorticoid release, as dexamethasone is able to reverse the effects of OXT on memory [28]. While OXT may facilitate memory and social interactions in certain contexts such as pair bonds at certain levels, robust levels of OXT may impair social memory due to substantial glucocorticoid release or impaired cholinergic activity.

3. Oxytocin in female animals

3.1. OXT and female animal affiliation

OXT mediates the establishment and support of social bonds in several female mammalian species. Central injection of OXT specifically facilitates pair bonding in female prairie voles, similar to the role of AVP in males [3, 29, 30]. Studies of OXT receptor distributions in voles have identified expression patterns linked to species patterns of social organization, which support the manipulative studies [5, 11]. It has been postulated that the role of OXT in female rodent affiliation may be related to its effects on maternal behavior [31]. In primates, affiliation has been correlated with urinary OXT levels, including a relationship between the solicitation of sex and increased OXT levels [9].

3.2. OXT and female animal aggression

The data on the role OXT in female aggression are mixed, including several studies specifically on maternal aggression [32]. Although it was initially concluded that OXT in the PVN had excitatory effects on maternal aggression [33, 34], more recent studies involving OXT manipulations in the CeA and BNST conclude that OXT has inhibitory effects on maternal aggression [35]. Other studies reporting a positive association between OXT and female aggression postulate that OXT increases aggression by attenuating fear [34, 36, 37], but it is also possible that elevated OXT levels following maternal aggression are a result of the stress of the encounter [36]. In contrast, maternal separation decreases OXT immunoreactivity in lactating female mice, and this decrease was associated with an decreased latency to attack a novel male intruder [38], supporting earlier studies reporting an inhibitory effect of OXT on maternal aggression [39-41]. Several studies of the effects of cocaine on maternal aggression and oxytocin have also concluded that oxytocin has inhibitory effects on aggression [42-44]. In multiparous rats which are more aggressive than primiparous dams, OXT or OXT receptor levels are decreased in several behaviorally relevant brain regions compared to primiparous animals [45]. In general, the majority of the manipulative studies support the conclusion that OXT is inhibitory towards female aggression.

3.3. OXT and animal maternal behavior

The importance of OXT in the establishment of maternal care was initially reported in the late 70's and early 80's through icv injections of OXT [46, 47], which have been supported by

OXT antagonist administration [48-50]. OXT receptor knockout mice exhibit deficits in maternal care [51]. However, central OXT activity may not be a factor in all aspects of maternal care. The initiation of maternal care is impaired by the disruption of central OXT activity by lesions and antagonism of OXT [11], but since OXT disrupting lesions to the PVN of sheep do not disrupt maternal care once it has been established, OXT appears to be more important in the initiation of maternal care than the maintenance [52]. Other investigations in sheep have supported the hypothesis that OXT specifically mediates the induction of maternal care [53]. Comprehensive studies of natural variations in rodent maternal care indicate that OXT receptors mediate these differences, with high levels of OXT activity being associated with elevated levels of maternal care [54, 55]. These OXT actions are related to associated changes in dopamine activity [56] and both OXT receptor levels and maternal care are altered by exposure to gestational stress [57]. It is postulated that impairments in maternal care following gestational stress may be mediated by decreases in central OXT activity. The actions of OXT receptors in the nucleus accumbens have also been implicated in spontaneous maternal care in prairie voles [58]. OXT's role in maternal care induction parallels the importance of this peptide in parturition and lactation, and there is clinical interest in these parallels. Future animal work which includes the behavioral and physiological effects of OXT in maternal animals may identify treatments for disorders involving deficits in both maternal care and lactation.

3.4. OXT in female animal models of depression and anxiety

Despite the established role of OXT in maternal care, a potent reward mediated behavior; little effort has been directed at studying the role of OXT in female depression and anxiety. Much of the current focus on translational OXT work is centered on effects on social behavior, and related disorders such as seasonal affective disorder and autism. Central OXT decreases anxiety in pregnant and lactating rats, despite having no effect in virgins [59]. However, chronic icv OXT is anxiolytic in female rats selected for high levels of anxiety [21]. Studies using ovariectomized rats indicate that circulating estrogen is required for the anxiolytic effects of OXT, which is likely to involve dynamic estrogen dependent changes in OXT receptor levels [60]. This dependence on estrogen may explain the divergent results in maternal and nulliparous rats considering the robust hormonal changes of pregnancy and lactation [61]. Elevated plus maze (EPM) testing indicates that the anxiolytic effects of OXT may be most potent in stressful context, as OXT is only anxiolytic when the EPM is presented as a novel environment [62]. These data are relevant to the clinical observation that exposure to stress is a significant predictor of depression in females [63]. The animal literature on OXT and maternal care and the consistency between animal and human work make this neuropeptide a strong target for human studies of postpartum depression.

3.5. OXT and female animal learning and memory

The majority of the studies on OXT and memory in female animals investigate social recognition. The disruption of endogenous OXT activity impairs short-term olfactory memory in female rats [64], and mice with a conditional OXT knockout display impairments in social recognition [65]. In sheep, a functioning OXT circuit in the olfactory bulb is required for offspring recognition [52]. These effects of OXT on offspring recognition are mediated by GABA, norepinephrine, and acetylcholine and are crucial to the role of OXT in maternal care induction [66]. It has also been postulated that the effects of OXT in pair bonding involve a social recognition function [67]. Similar to studies of the roles of dopamine and AVP in rodent maternal memory (the ability of a dam to quickly return to maternal care following a separation from her pups) [68, 69], central OXT is involved in the consolidation of maternal memory [70]. One hypothesis is that the effects of both OXT and AVP are mediated by their actions on dopamine. Although some studies of ongoing maternal care conclude that OXT is not necessary once offspring care has been established [11, 52, 71], these data on maternal memory indicate that its importance to maternal care may extend beyond the initial stages of maternal care.

4. Oxytocin in male humans

4.1. OXT and male human affiliation

The investigations of OXT and affiliation in humans do not necessarily examine affiliation directly. For instance, intranasal OXT promotes trust and prosocial behaviors which are critical to human bonding and it is also associated with trustworthiness [72, 73]. Intranasal OXT increases cooperation following unreciprocated cooperation in a social experiment and this behavioral effect was associated with increased fMRI activity in OXT regions associated with affiliation [74]. Studies investigating affiliation and/or sexual behavior conclude that the effects of OXT are often mediated by direct physical contact as increased plasma OXT has been recorded in men during social contact with a partner [75], and during orgasm [76-78].

Impaired affiliation has been associated with decreased plasma OXT in autistic patients [79]. Normal affiliative expression is especially impaired in autistic males, and some autistic males have deficits in OXT receptor expression [80, 81]. Several cases were associated with hypermethylation of the OXT receptor gene and a decrease in OXT receptor mRNA. Furthermore, clinical studies have reported enhanced social interactions (eye contact, social memory) in autistic patients following intranasal OXT [82]. Several labs have investigated the use of OXT for the treatment of social behavior deficits in autism [82-84] and social anxiety disorder [85], and research in this area is ongoing.

4.2. OXT and male human aggression

Compared to the interest in OXT and human prosocial behavior, there are few studies of the role of OXT on male aggression. The established effects on affiliation and prosocial behavior in animals and humans support the hypothesis that OXT has inhibitory effects on aggression. Conversely, some have postulated that OXT's anxiolytic effects could result in increased aggression, but there are no behavioral data in support of this theory. One potential clinical role of OXT is in the treatment of PTSD associated aggression.

4.3. OXT and human paternal behavior

There is some evidence that OXT mediates human paternal care as well as maternal care. Plasma and salivary OXT has been associated with paternal social engagement, affect synchrony, and positive communication sequences, and fathers who exhibit high levels of stimulatory contact with 4-6 month old infants have elevated OXT levels compared to fathers that do not exhibit high levels of contact [86]. Intranasal OXT increases the responsiveness of fathers during play with their children, and may decrease hostility, which supports a causal role for OXT and positive paternal behavior [87]. The decrease in hostility offers indirect support for an inhibitory effect on male aggression. Finally, both maternal and paternal plasma OXT levels predict coordination of behaviors between parents and their children, indicating that OXT may have a positive effect on family interactions [88, 89]. Collectively, these recent studies indicate that OXT modulates several forms of family associated social behavior.

4.4. OXT and male human depression and anxiety

The interest in OXT as a potential treatment for mood disorders is based on the animal literature supporting the involvement of OXT in reward mediated and social behaviors [90, 91], which are often impaired in depressed individuals. Reduced plasma OXT has been observed in humans suffering from depression [92, 93], and detailed investigations of depressive symptoms indicate that high levels of plasma OXT are associated with a decrease in the severity of symptoms [94]. However, some studies have been unable to find depression related differences in plasma OXT [95]. Since OXT has both central behavioral effects and peripheral physiological effects, the exact functions of elevated plasma OXT are not clear. The few studies which have measured OXT activity in postmortem samples of depressed patients have reported increases in depression associated OXT immunoreactivity [96] and OXT mRNA in the PVN [97]. The increase in OXT mRNA in melancholic patients compared to non-melancholic depressives suggests that changes in OXT are specific to the type of depression. With anxiety, intranasal OXT has minor effects in male patients with seasonal affective disorder [85]. Given the strength of the animal work on the prosocial and reward mediated actions of OXT, it is surprising that there is not more interest in this target for treating depression and/or anxiety.

4.5. OXT and male human learning and memory

Intranasal OXT facilitates socially reinforced learning and emotional empathy in men [98], consistent with the data from animal models and the initial studies of the effects of OXT in autistic patients. Another study reported that OXT's effects were specific to the social stimuli of facial expressions, and did not affect financial associations in an associative learning task [99]. The available evidence supports the conclusion that OXT facilitates social reinforced learning and memory in human males, and these effects may be mediated at the amygdala [98].

5. Oxytocin in female humans

5.1. OXT and female human affiliation

OXT levels in females rise during massage, genital stimulation, copulation, and orgasm [11, 100] which parallels the association between OXT and physical contact in men. In a study of intrapersonal couple conflict, intranasal OXT increases positive communication and decreases plasma cortisol [101]. It is suggested that OXT may facilitate pair bonding in humans, as in voles. Women with more supportive partners have increased OXT before, during, and after a 10 minute period of physical contact [75]. In contrast, OXT is positively correlated with interpersonal conflict [102, 103], but the relevance of these changes in OXT is debated [104]. This increase in OXT may be in response to the conflict and not a causal factor. Some have speculated that plasma OXT may be a reliable biomarker of distressed relationships in female humans [105]. Intranasal OXT alters the neural response to emotional faces in women, and these effects differ from the effects in males (Domes 2010). One hypothesis is that OXT increases as a mechanism to ameliorate the negative effect of the conflict on the social bond, but further manipulative studies are needed in this area.

5.2. OXT and human maternal behavior

OXT is an important mediator of maternal-infant bonding in humans [106]. Increasing OXT during pregnancy is associated with enhanced maternal bonding [107]. Maternal behaviors such as gazing at the infant, touching, and attachment related thoughts are associated with OXT levels in both early pregnancy and postpartum periods [108]. Mothers who display high levels of affectionate contact exhibit an increase in plasma and salivary OXT, while similar increases are not exhibited by mothers displaying low levels of contact [86]. The primary importance of OXT in human maternal behavior appears to be in enhancing bonding during the first few weeks of lactation [71, 109]. Furthermore, mothers viewing images of their own infants increase brain activity in reward nuclei that contain high levels of OXT and AVP receptors [110]. In breastfeeding women, basal OXT levels are negatively correlated with anxiety and guilt [111], and plasma OXT in mothers is also associated with affectionate touch between mothers, fathers, and offspring [88]. It is concluded that OXT is an important mediator of the formation and maintenance of the family unit. Mothers that may have less efficient OXT systems display lower levels of sensitive responsiveness to their 2 year old toddlers [112]. Intranasal OXT treated mothers use less handgrip force in response to infant cry sounds, but this effect is only present in mothers who were not harshly disciplined as children [113]. One explanation for these effects is that high levels of early life discipline have developmental effects on central OXT circuits which make these individuals less responsive to exogenous OXT. In mothers who used cocaine during pregnancy, decreased OXT levels were associated with greater hostility and depressed mood, results consistent with animal studies reporting inhibitory effects of OXT on aggression. These mothers were also less likely to hold their babies, suggesting impaired bonding [114]. In a fMRI study, securely attached mothers exhibited a more robust OXT response to images of their own infants when crying and smiling, and also had increased neural responses in brain regions association with reward, such as the ventral striatum [115]. Most notably, it has recently been reported that low plasma OXT concentrations during pregnancy are associated with an increased risk for postpartum depression. Plasma OXT concentrations in mid pregnancy significantly predicted PPD symptoms at 2 weeks postpartum [116]. Taken together, the data on OXT and maternal behavior strongly support the targeting of central OXT in the development of new treatments for maternal mood disorders.

5.3. OXT and female human depression and anxiety

Although plasma OXT is difficult to measure and has a high degree of variability, reduced plasma OXT has been documented in both males and females suffering from depression [117]. Changes in the variability of OXT pulses have also been reported in women with major depression [118]. Given the gender differences reported for the roles of AVP and OXT in animal studies, it is likely that there are neuroendocrine differences in the role of OXT and AVP in human depression as well. Studies of maternal humans suggest that OXT may be specifically involved in the development of postpartum mood disorders. Women with lower plasma OXT while interacting with their own infants are at an increased risk for depression due to low attachment ratings as adults and low attachment ratings for their children [115]. Cocaine addicted mothers, who are at an increased risk for postpartum mood disorders which result in impaired maternal infant attachment also have depressed plasma OXT levels [114]. Childhood trauma, which is a reliable predictor of adult depression, has been associated with decreased CSF OXT and high levels of anxiety [119, 120]. Both prior stressful events and current exposure to stress are significant predictors of postpartum depression, so the association between stress and OXT may be involved in a common mechanism for the development of postpartum mood disorders. As mentioned previously, low plasma OXT during pregnancy predicts an increased risk for postpartum depression [116] and elevated OXT in postpartum women is associated with low levels of anxiety [111]. The advantage of targeting clinical studies of OXT and depression at postpartum depression is that improvements in these patients is also beneficial to the rest of the family, and may represent a preventative target for the offspring of depressed mothers. Furthermore, there has been recent speculation that failed lactation and perinatal depression have related neuroendocrine mechanisms [121]. Failed lactation is common in depressed mothers, and in many cases can exacerbate symptoms of depression in mothers.

5.4. OXT and female human learning and memory

The strongest support for a role of OXT in human memory is found in studies of affiliation. Social bonds require memory related components of social recognition. It is postulated that OXT's role in bonding involves social recognition and memory mechanisms [122]. Studies from male subjects suggest that despite a potential amnesiac function of OXT in certain paradigms, central OXT may enhance social memory [123]. It is unknown whether OXT has similar effects in women.

6. AVP in male animals

6.1. AVP and male animal affiliation

There is a wealth of studies of AVP and affiliation in voles [11]. Central administration of AVP to monogamous prairie voles that live in burrows with extended families induces several forms of bonding behaviors [124, 125], and AVP V1a receptor antagonist treatment blocks pair bonding behaviors in males [124, 125]. In polygamous montane voles (*Microtus montanus*) that live in solitary burrows, AVP or V1a antagonist treatments have no effects on social behavior. These behavioral differences are reflected in the neural OXT and AVP maps of these species [5]. Over-expression of V1a receptors in the forebrain of male prairie voles enhances pair bonding [126], and V1a antagonist injection into specific brain regions inhibit pair bond formation [127, 128]. The pattern of AVP mediated pair bonding in males and OXT mediated pair bonding in females has been identified in several other species [129]. Although there is no clear picture of how AVP expression patterns relate to social structure, AVP is an important mediator of affiliation in many vertebrate species, including fish [2] and birds [1]. The variety of social structures and central AVP circuitry among vertebrate species presents a valuable opportunity for both descriptive and manipulative comparative studies.

6.2. AVP and male animal aggression

Initial studies in male hamsters reported that V1a antagonist administration into the anterior hypothalamus inhibits aggression [130, 131], results which have since been confirmed in several other labs [132-134]. Exogenous AVP in the anterior hypothalamus can stimulate offensive aggression [133, 135], but this effect may be modulated by social environment [136]. Further work in hamsters has revealed that an orally active V1a antagonist decreases aggression in male hamsters, but does not affect social investigation or sexual motivation [137]. Anabolic steroid treatment of adolescent males increases aggression which can be inhibited by V1a antagonist treatment in the AH [138], indicating that the elevated aggression is mediated by central AVP activity. A similar effect of amphetamine has been documented in male prairie voles, where increased aggression is associated with increased V1a receptor binding in the AH [134]. Developmental effects of AVP have been reported in male prairie voles, where early postnatal peripheral injections of AVP increase adult aggression [139]. However, maternal separation in mice increases AVP in the paraventricular nucleus and decreases intermale aggression [38]. This effect is similar to much of the behavioral data from female animals, which indicate that AVP has suppressive effects on maternal aggression and intraspecies aggression.

6.3. AVP and animal paternal behavior

Research on AVP and offspring care by males includes studies in several rodent species. The increase in paternal behavior in cohabitating meadow voles is mediated by AVP, as treatment with AVP antagonist decreases paternal behavior [14, 140]. Elevated AVP in meadow voles stimulates paternal behavior through both a decrease in pup directed aggression and an increase in paternal behaviors [14]. Alloparental behavior in naïve male prairie voles also involves central AVP actions [15]. Monogamous male California mice are more paternal and aggressive towards nest intruders than polygamous male while footed mice, and these differences are associated with elevated AVP in the BNST and LS [141]. These paternal styles may be transmitted through behavioral effects, as cross-fostering paternal behavior is similar to the foster parent behavior [142]. Pup directed aggression may be decreased and paternal care increased through social bonding mediated changes in central AVP. It is likely that the effects of AVP on paternal behavior are related to its general role in social bonding.

6.4. AVP and male animal models of depression and anxiety

Anxiety related behavior on the elevated plus maze is decreased following septal AVP antagonist treatment or antisense treatment in male rats [143, 144]. In contrast, other studies report that intraseptal and intraperitoneal AVP is anxiolytic [145]. An anxiogenic role of AVP is supported by male AVP V1a receptor knockout mice which exhibit lower levels of anxiety compared to wild type [24, 146]. Once again, other investigations of this line have failed to find differences in anxiety [147]. The oral and intraperitoneal administration of an AVP V1b antagonist is anxiolytic in several tests of anxiety [148-150], but AVP V1b receptor knockout males may not exhibit decreased anxiety [147, 151]. The lack of differences in anxiety related behaviors in these knockout mice may be due to compensatory mechanisms during development. In male rats bred for high levels of anxiety, AVP level and release from the PVN are elevated when compared to low anxiety males [152-154] and the differential expression of AVP in rats selected for high anxiety has been linked to specific single nucleotide polymorphisms [155, 156]. Central AVP V1a receptor antagonist treatment decreases anxiety and depression associated behaviors in high anxiety males [154]. The forced swim test induces both depression associated behavior and elevated AVP in the SON and PVN [157, 158]. V1a antagonist treatment to both the mediolateral septum and amygdala has antidepressant like effects in male animals [159, 160], and similar effects are documented following V1b receptor antagonist treatment [148, 161]. For male animals, there is evidence to support the hypothesis that depression and anxiety related behaviors are associated with elevated AVP activity in both brain and plasma.

6.5. AVP and male animal learning and memory

Infusion of AVP into the lateral septum of wild type and AVP deficient Brattleboro rats enhances social memory, and these effects are impaired by antagonist or antisense treatments [162, 163]. The over expression of vole V1a receptors in rats enhances social discrimination abilities [164]. However, studies of V1a and V1b KO mice have had mixed results, with some reporting impaired social recognition [24, 151] and others failing to find impairments [165]. AVP has also been implicated in both memory consolidation [166] and memory retrieval [167, 168]. The social aspects of AVP's effect on memory suggest the roles of this nonapeptide in memory and affiliation are related.

7. AVP in female animals

7.1. AVP and female animal affiliation

Most of the work on AVP and pairbonding in voles has focused on the male vole. Several studies indicate that OXT is more important than AVP for female pair bonding [169]. It is known that OXT receptor and AVP V1a antagonists prevent pair bond formation in both males and females [170]. Studies of AVP and maternal behavior indirectly support the hypothesis that AVP is a mediator of female affiliation [48, 171], but it is unknown if these effects pertain to adult conspecific affiliation. Additional studies on females are needed to determine if central AVP also is a significant mediator of the female component of pairbonding.

7.2. AVP and female animal aggression

Several studies have reported that AVP has inhibitory effects on maternal aggression towards a male intruder, which contrasts with the stimulatory role of AVP in male rodent aggression. V1a antagonist treatment increases maternal aggression in both primiparous and multiparous dams, and AVP injection decreases maternal aggression in highly aggressive multiparous rats [171, 172]. An inhibitory role for AVP in females is also supported by multiple experiments in non-maternal female hamsters [173]. Gene expression analysis of primiparous and multiparous rats indicates that changes in both AVP and OXT may be involved in the parity associated increase in maternal aggression in multiparous rats, as high levels of aggression are associated with low levels of AVP and OXT activity in several nuclei [45]. fMRI study of the neural effects of V1a antagonist treatment during the presentation of a novel male intruder reveal that this treatment may increase aggressive responding by enhancing the somatosensory responses to a male intruder and reducing fear responses in the cortical amygdala and ventromedial hypothalamus [174]. One hypothesis derived from these data is that AVP increases the perceived threat from the male intruder. Although some studies have found increased AVP release associated with maternal aggression, it is hypothesized that this release is triggered by the stressful nature of the encounter [36]. Manipulations of AVP in rat strains selected for anxiety behaviors reveal an excitatory function of AVP on aggression, but this effect on aggression only involves behavioral frequencies, and it is not known if the decreased frequencies are associated with increased durations of aggressive bouts [175].

7.3. AVP and animal maternal behavior

Recent studies indicate that OXT is not the only nonapeptide involved in the modulation of mammalian maternal care. Both AVP and V1a antagonist treatments decrease maternal care during exposure to a male intruder, with the effects of AVP associated with increased self grooming and the effects of V1a antagonist associated with elevated maternal aggression during resident intruder tests of maternal aggression [171]. Studies focusing specifically on maternal care conclude that central AVP promotes ongoing maternal care [48]. Furthermore, the blockade of V1a receptors around parturition impairs maternal memory, the ability of a maternal dam to return to maternal care following a prolonged separation from her pups [68]. Although it has been postulated that maternal nurturing is linked to innate anxiety and OXT and AVP activity, this is based mostly on studies of rodent lines selected for anxiety [175]. Low anxiety mice display lower levels of maternal care compared to high anxiety mice, and acute icv injection of AVP increases maternal care and has anxiogenic effects [176]. These effects in mice were only moderately attenuated by cross fostering. An association between maternal care and innate anxiety was not supported in another study of maternal mice, although V1a receptors were correlated with pup grooming [177]. Animal studies suggest that AVP may be a worthwhile target for the development of treatments for anxiety associated disorders that affect maternal behavior, such as postpartum depression, which is often comorbid with anxiety.

7.4. AVP and female animal models of depression and anxiety

Many of the mechanistic studies of AVP and depression and anxiety have focused on males, and there is a need for more detailed studies in both nulliparous and pregnant and maternal females. As mentioned in the maternal behavior section, high anxiety rats and mice have elevated AVP activity in the PVN and display increased anxiety and depression behaviors [31, 176]. However, recent studies on a novel social stress mediated model for postpartum depression suggest that AVP can increase maternal care in animals subjected to the social stress paradigm that attenuates maternal care and aggression and impairs dam and pup growth during lactation [220]. At the present time, much of the available data on AVP and maternal behavior conflicts with the depression data from males, and treatments with V1a/V1b antagonists aimed at decreasing anxiety may have negative effects on maternal care.

7.5. AVP and female animal learning and memory

The little work that has focused on AVP and female memory has predominately used pregnant or maternal females. Female V1b knockout mice do not display the Bruce effect, where a previously mated female will block the implantation of fertilized eggs if exposed to an unfamiliar male after mating [178]. This suggests that the female's long-term social memory is impaired. As noted in the maternal behavior section, a V1a antagonist around parturition impairs the ability of a dam to re-initiate maternal care [68]. In general, the available data on AVP and female memory supports the literature from males concluding that AVP mediates various forms of memory consolidation and retention and has particular relevance to social memory. If the role of AVP in memory is substantial in human females, it is possible that depression and anxiety treatments targeted at antagonizing central AVP may impair memory processes.

8. AVP in male humans

8.1. AVP and male human affiliation

Intranasal AVP has been reported to enhance the encoding of emotional facial expressions in humans [179], as well as improving the recognition of sexual cues [180]. Other studies indicate that intranasal AVP increases the negative emotional response to neutral facial expressions [181, 182]. These effects appear to be gender specific, as intranasal AVP in men stimulates agonistic responses to the faces of novel men, but stimulates affiliative facial responses in women and increases positive perceptions of these faces [181]. AVP increases cooperative behavior in men in response to a cooperative gesture in a social experiment, and this behavioral effect was associated with fMRI activity in brain regions involved in affiliative responses [74]. It has been suggested that plasma AVP may be a biomarker of distressed relationships in men [105]. Similar to several other behavioral topics, these gender specific effects need to be considered with respect to treatment development.

8.2. AVP and male human aggression

AVP levels in cerebrospinal fluid (csf) have been correlated with aggression in male humans [183]. However, a study comparing csf AVP in violent offenders vs. controls found no differences [184]. Patients with PTSD often have difficulties controlling their aggression levels, and clinical studies suggest that plasma levels are elevated in war veterans with PTSD [185]. Furthermore, intranasal AVP enhances physiological responding to combat images in male Vietnam veterans compared to saline and OXT [186], and AVP has been identified as a likely mediator for the effects of early life stress on the development of PTSD [187]. The available clinical evidence supports continued investigation of central AVP in the development of treatments for aggression disorders.

8.3. AVP and male human depression and anxiety

The first study suggesting that AVP was involved in mood disorders was from 1978 [188]. Plasma AVP is elevated in male patients with depression [95], and it has been suggested that increased AVP mRNA in the SON mediates the elevated plasma AVP levels [97]. Some have hypothesized that plasma AVP is specifically correlated to melancholic depression [97] as well as suicide [189, 190]. In terms of the prevalence of depression within a population, elevated plasma AVP is correlated with anxiety and a family history of depression [191, 192]. Resilience against depression has been associated with a SNP of the V1b receptor gene [193]. These data have generated continued interest in AVP antagonists in the treatment of mood disorders [194, 195].

8.4. AVP and male human learning and memory

Administration of an AVP analog enhances memory in human males [196, 197]. Treatment of boys with learning disorders with acute or chronic AVP increases the ability to remember stories. However, synthetic AVP may only affect reaction time, not memory [198]. In elderly humans, however, repeated intranasal AVP does not improve long term memory [199]. One hypothesis is that the memory enhancing effects of AVP are mediated by a general increase in arousal [200], although animal work suggests that AVP has specific effects on the molecular mechanisms of long term memory consolidation [201, 202].

9. AVP in female humans

9.1. AVP and female human affiliation

In contrast to the pro-aggressive effects of intranasal AVP in men, AVP induces affiliative facial motor patterns in women in response to the faces of unfamiliar women and increases the perception of the faces as friendly. This gender specific effect supports the animal work on AVP. In contrast, the AVP treatment increased anxiety in both sexes [181]. Homozygosity for the RS3 allele 334 doubles the risk of marital difficulties, and negatively influenced how the relationship was perceived by the spouse [203]. Central AVP activity may be a worthwhile target for gender specific treatments aimed at improving human pair bonds.

9.2. AVP and human maternal behavior

Studies of multiparous humans report that maternal sensitivity is associated with the AVP V1a receptor gene. Mothers with 2 copies of the long RS3 alleles were less sensitive than mothers with one or zero copies of the long allele, and this association was most prevalent in mothers exposed to high maternal adversity [204]. A valid question is how this polymorphism affects affiliation in females, as in the Walum et al. 2008 study. Exposure to maternal neglect is associated with depressed urinary AVP levels in children [205]. The effects were persistent despite being in a stable environment for three years following the maternal neglect. It was concluded that social deprivation inhibits the long-term development of the central AVP system, and this effect may be involved in the etiology of neglect associated mood disorders.

9.3. AVP and female human female depression and anxiety

Much of the research on this topic is focused on the interaction between stress, AVP, and depression. Specific V1b receptor haplotypes are associated with protection against recurrent major depression in both males and females [193]. A more recent study has found the association between V1b gene variants, AVP single nucleotide polymorphisms (SNP's), and vulnerability to childhood onset depression in females [206, 207]. In a study of male and female depression patients, plasma AVP was highly correlated with depression in non-treated patients, but this correlation was not found in patients taking anti-depressants [191]. These studies suggest that the central AVP system is a valid target for treatments for depression and anxiety.

10. Translation from animals to humans

10.1. Stress

There is a great deal of translational overlap in the research areas where focus on AVP and OXT is most relevant, and this is especially true with the studies on the effects of stress. Exposure to acute and/or chronic stress is often a predictor of depression/anxiety, addiction relapse, and relationship difficulties. It is suggested that the most valuable paradigms for investigating the roles of AVP and OXT in depression, anxiety, or addiction involve exposure to chronic stress. The use of ethologically relevant stressors in animal models, such as social stress, is most likely to produce translationally consistent results (effects in animals which parallel clinical data). Many commonly used chronic stress protocols used in studies of AVP/OXT and depression and anxiety, such as chronic mild stress, do not use stressors associated with human disorders.

While the role of AVP in the endocrine stress response has been studied in detail at the animal level, the effects of stress on OXT are not as well known. Integrative investigations which include both AVP and OXT may indentify novel interactions between these behaviorally potent peptides. The most promising translational area may be PTSD. There is already evidence that male PTSD patients have high plasma AVP, aggression, depression and anxiety levels and similar behavioral effects have been associated with elevated AVP in animals. While it is difficult to separate the changes in depression and anxiety from impairments in social behavior, an increased focus on OXT in PTSD studies may provide insight on the social deficits in PTSD patients. Social bonds are often negatively impacted by exposure to chronic stress, and these bonds can have a positive buffering effect on the negative effects of chronic stress.

An indication of the potential value of social support can be seen in the cultural comparison of postpartum depression prevalence. Societies that have high levels of social support for mothers have low rates of depression, and cultures with low levels of support have much higher rates [208]. There is evidence that social support has protective effects in stress related mood disorders, and understanding the role of AVP and OXT in the positive effects of social support may help maximize the value of social support focused interventions.

10.2. Depression and anxiety

Increases the prevalence of stress related mood disorders [209] combined with metanalyses reporting that current treatments for depression may not be effective for mild to moderate depression [210] make a compelling argument that a new approach is needed in depression and anxiety research. Both the animal and human studies suggest that AVP is involved in the development of depression and anxiety disorders, and several reports indicate that AVP has gender specific roles. Continuing development of AVP targeted treatments should consider these gender specific actions. It is possible that while V1a antagonists may work for alleviating depression and/or anxiety symptoms in males, AVP or AVP agonists may be more effective in females. As noted by Manning et al. there has been little success with the development of non-peptide agonists and antagonists for AVP despite substantial investments by pharmaceutical companies. In contrast, some progress has been made with OXT peptide based treatments [194, 195]. The recent studies on AVP and maternal behavior in animals suggest that increased focus on AVP in human studies is warranted, especially on stress, maternal behavior, and postpartum depression. One valuable use for non-peptide ligands that have not been successful in clinical trials is as research tools, including the development of specific AVP and OXT ligands for imaging studies [194].

The animal and human data on OXT support the hypothesis that this peptide hormone is also a valid target for novel maternal mood disorder treatments. An interesting implication in this area is that synthetic OXT is already commonly used to induce labor, yet little is known about how this treatment may affect maternal behavior and/or offspring. OXT or OXT antagonists may also be effective in treating melancholic depression and seasonal affective disorder. There are also interesting non-pharmaceutical interventions which can manipulate OXT levels, such as physical touch and modified birthing practices and procedures (cesarean sections and induced labor vs. natural childbirth). Greater collaboration between animal and clinical researchers will accelerate the development of safe and effective AVP and OXT targeted treatments for depression and anxiety disorders, including postpartum depression, seasonal affective disorder, and PTSD. Projects that involve consistent interactions between animal and clinical researchers throughout the developmental process will be most effective. Another potential therapeutic application of AVP and OXT is in relationship counseling. Both of these hormones are likely to be involved in the mechanisms of establishing and maintaining the social bond necessary for a strong and stable relationship. AVP and OXT targeted treatments may be effective in treating the adverse effects of chronic social conflict, or the effects of other chronic stressors, especially in combination with behavioral cognitive therapy.

10.3. Addiction

Both affiliative behavior and addiction are mediated through similar central reward pathways. Central OXT pathways are also altered by addiction. Endogenous OXT activity is suppressed by chronic drug use, and elevated brain OXT levels may attenuate the negative effects of withdrawal [211]. There is preliminary evidence that exogenous OXT is capable of inhibiting stimulant and alcohol self administration and it may prevent stress and priming induced relapse [212]. As with autism, OXT centered treatments may be a useful adjunct to behavioral cognitive techniques. For example, intranasal OXT may augment the positive effects of extinction training for addiction [213] and/or reduce rates of relapse.

Levels of AVP mRNA increase in the amygdala during early withdrawal from cocaine [214], and the blockade of V1b receptors can block reinstatement in rodents [215]. In a rodent model of ethanol dependence, a V1b antagonist decreases excessive levels of ethanol self administration [216]. There is further evidence that AVP secretion is attenuated in response to social stress in the sons of alcohol dependent fathers, but it is unclear how these results relate to the risk of developing an addiction [217]. While data from humans is lacking, the involvement of AVP in the etiology of stress related depression and anxiety suggests that this hormone may be implicated in the long term effects of addiction and the mechanisms mediating relapse. V1b antagonism may be a productive translational target for not only drug dependence, but addiction associated depression and anxiety as well.

10.4. Autism

While current translational efforts with OXT and autism acknowledge that the effectiveness of intranasal OXT treatments may only be relevant to social behavior deficits, the animal studies of AVP/OXT on learning suggest that there may be additional benefits to focusing translational studies in this area. One animal research topic that may be of particular interest is the developmental role of AVP and OXT. Treatments which only affect social behavior in older children or adults may be effective with other impairments when administered at a younger age. Changes in the brains of autistic children have been observed in children as young as 6 months [218]. Another issue with the current clinical trials of intranasal oxytocin is the level of dosing. There is debate as to how much OXT crosses the blood brain barrier and has central effects. One hypothesis is that developmental AVP manipulation may be able to address the cognitive impairments of autism. While most of the clinical efforts in AVP/OXT and autism are centered on the development of pharmaceutical treatments, environmental changes may also be effective. It is possible that insults during gestation, such as chronic social stress, are affecting the normal development of AVP/OXT mediated cognitive and social pathways. Another potential benefit of an OXT focused therapy may be as an adjunct to behavioral therapies aimed at improving social skills. One of the limitations of the current OXT manipulations is the available administration methods. The prairie vole partner preference model is a valuable tool for the screening of novel OXT treatments and administration methods [219].

11. Conclusions

In summary, increased translation between the animal research and clinical studies in males and females on the social behavior roles of AVP and OXT has the potential to stimulate rapid progress in the development of effective treatments for stress related disorders, including PTSD, depression and anxiety, and addiction, as well as disorders which involve deficits in affiliation, such as autism. These treatments may involve pharmalogical interventions, modifications to current practices, social interventions, or a combination of approaches. Stress paradigms which are ethologically relevant to both animals and humans, such as social stress for studies of depression and addiction, may generate the most useful data. PTSD and postpartum depression are two disorders that may benefit greatly from AVP and OXT focused studies. Given the available literature on the substantial gender differences in the roles of AVP and OXT, continued research on these peptide hormones needs to include studies of both males and females.

Author details

Benjamin C. Nephew
Department of Biomedical Sciences, Tufts University Cummings School of Veterinary Medicine, North Grafton, MA, USA

12. References

[1] Goodson, J.L., A.M. Kelly, and M.A. Kingsbury, *Evolving nonapeptide mechanisms of gregariousness and social diversity in birds.* Hormones and Behavior, 2012. 61(3): p. 239-250.

[2] Godwin, J. and R. Thompson, *Nonapeptides and Social Behavior in Fishes.* Hormones and Behavior, 2012. 61(3): p. 230-238.

[3] Williams, J.R., T.R. Insel, C.R. Harbaugh, and C.S. Carter, *Oxytocin administered centrally facilitates formation of a partner preference in prairie voles (Microtus ochrogaster).* J. Neuroendocrinol., 1994. 6: p. 247-250.

[4] Bales, K. and C.S. Carter, *Developmental exposure to oxytocin facilitates partner preferences in male prairie voles (Microtus ochrogaster).* Behav. Neurosci., 2003. 117: p. 854-859.

[5] Insel, T.R. and L.E. Shapiro, *Oxytocin receptor distribution reflects social organization in monogamous and polygamous voles.* Proc. Natl. Acad. Sci. USA, 1992. 89: p. 5981-5985.

[6] Ferguson, J., L. Young, E. Hearn, M. Matzuk, T. Insel, and J. Winslow, *Social amnesia in mice lacking the oxytocin gene.* Nat Genet, 2000. 25: p. 284 - 288.

[7] Ferguson, J.N., J.M. Aldag, T.R. Insel, and L.J. Young, *Oxytocin in the medial amygdala is essential for social recognition in the mouse.* J. Neurosci., 2001. 21: p. 8278-8285.

[8] Witt, D.M. and T.R. Insel, *Increased Fos Expression in Oxytocin Neurons Following Masculine Sexual Behavior.* Journal of Neuroendocrinology, 1994. 6(1): p. 13-18.

[9] Snowdon, C.T., B.A. Pieper, C.Y. Boe, K.A. Cronin, A.V. Kurian, and T.E. Ziegler, *Variation in oxytocin is related to variation in affiliative behavior in monogamous, pairbonded tamarins.* Hormones and Behavior, 2010. 58(4): p. 614-618.

[10] Kleszczyńska, A., E. Sokołowska, and E. Kulczykowska, *Variation in brain arginine vasotocin (AVT) and isotocin (IT) levels with reproductive stage and social status in males of three-spined stickleback (Gasterosteus aculeatus).* General and Comparative Endocrinology, 2012. 175(2): p. 290-296.

[11] Insel, T.R. and L.J. Young, *Neuropeptides and the evolution of social behavior.* Current Opinion in Neurobiology, 2000. 10(6): p. 784-789.

[12] DeVries, A.C., W.S. Young Iii, and R.J. Nelson, *Reduced Aggressive Behaviour in Mice with Targeted Disruption of the Oxytocin Gene.* Journal of Neuroendocrinology, 1997. 9(5): p. 363-368.

[13] Winslow, J. and T. Insel, *The social deficits of the oxytocin knockout mouse.* Neuropeptides, 2002. 36: p. 221 - 229.

[14] Parker, K.J., L.F. Kinney, K.M. Phillips, and T.M. Lee, *Paternal behavior is associated with central neurohormone receptor binding patterns in meadow voles (Microtus pennsylvanicus).* Behavioral Neuroscience, 2001. 115(6): p. 1341-1348.

[15] Bales, K.L., A.L. Kim, A.D. Lewis-Reese, and C.S. Carter, *Both oxytocin and vasopressin may influence alloparental behavior in male prairie voles.* Horm. Behav., 2004. 45: p. 354-361.

[16] Song, Z., F. Tai, C. Yu, R. Wu, X. Zhang, H. Broders, F. He, and R. Guo, *Sexual or paternal experiences alter alloparental behavior and the central expression of ERα and OT in male mandarin voles (Microtus mandarinus).* Behavioural Brain Research, 2010. 214(2): p. 290-300.

[17] Saito, A. and K. Nakamura, *Oxytocin changes primate paternal tolerance to offspring in food transfer.* Journal of Comparative Physiology A: Neuroethology, Sensory, Neural, and Behavioral Physiology, 2011. 197(4): p. 329-337.

[18] Arletti, R., A. Benelli, R. Poggioli, P. Luppi, B. Menozzi, and A. Bertolini, *Aged rats are still responsive to the antidepressant and memory-improving effects of oxytocin.* Neuropeptides, 1995. 29(3): p. 177-182.

[19] Arletti, R. and A. Bertolini, *Oxytocin acts as an antidepressant in two animal models of depression.* Life Sciences, 1987. 41(14): p. 1725-1730.

[20] Ring, R.H., L.E. Schechter, S.K. Leonard, J.M. Dwyer, B.J. Platt, R. Graf, S. Grauer, C. Pulicicchio, L. Resnick, Z. Rahman, S.J. Sukoff Rizzo, B. Luo, C.E. Beyer, S.F. Logue, K.L. Marquis, Z.A. Hughes, and S. Rosenzweig-Lipson, *Receptor and behavioral pharmacology of WAY-267464, a non-peptide oxytocin receptor agonist.* Neuropharmacology, 2010. 58(1): p. 69-77.

[21] Slattery, D.A. and I.D. Neumann, *Chronic icv oxytocin attenuates the pathological high anxiety state of selectively bred Wistar rats.* Neuropharmacology, 2010. 58(1): p. 56-61.

[22] Grippo, A.J., D. Gerena, J. Huang, N. Kumar, M. Shah, R. Ughreja, and C. Sue Carter, *Social isolation induces behavioral and neuroendocrine disturbances relevant to depression in female and male prairie voles.* Psychoneuroendocrinology, 2007. 32(8–10): p. 966-980.

[23] De Wied, D., *Behavioural Actions of Neurohypophysial Peptides.* Proceedings of the Royal Society of London. Series B. Biological Sciences, 1980. 210(1178): p. 183-194.

[24] Bielsky, I.F., S.B. Hu, K.L. Szegda, H. Westphal, and L.J. Young, *Profound impairment in social recognition and reduction in anxiety in vasopressin V1a receptor knockout mice.* Neuropsychopharmacology, 2004. 29: p. 483-493.

[25] Jin, D., H.-X. Liu, H. Hirai, T. Torashima, T. Nagai, O. Lopatina, N.A. Shnayder, K. Yamada, M. Noda, T. Seike, K. Fujita, S. Takasawa, S. Yokoyama, K. Koizumi, Y. Shiraishi, S. Tanaka, M. Hashii, T. Yoshihara, K. Higashida, M.S. Islam, N. Yamada, K. Hayashi, N. Noguchi, I. Kato, H. Okamoto, A. Matsushima, A. Salmina, T. Munesue, N. Shimizu, S. Mochida, M. Asano, and H. Higashida, *CD38 is critical for social behaviour by regulating oxytocin secretion.* Nature, 2007. 446(7131): p. 41-45.

[26] Boccia, M.M., S.R. Kopf, and C.M. Baratti, *Effects of a Single Administration of Oxytocin or Vasopressin and Their Interactions with Two Selective Receptor Antagonists on Memory Storage in Mice.* Neurobiology of Learning and Memory, 1998. 69(2): p. 136-146.

[27] Boccia, M.M. and C.M. Baratti, *Involvement of Central Cholinergic Mechanisms in the Effects of Oxytocin and an Oxytocin Receptor Antagonist on Retention Performance in Mice.* Neurobiology of Learning and Memory, 2000. 74(3): p. 217-228.

[28] de Oliveira, L.F., C. Camboim, F. Diehl, A.R. Consiglio, and J.A. Quillfeldt, *Glucocorticoid-mediated effects of systemic oxytocin upon memory retrieval.* Neurobiology of Learning and Memory, 2007. 87(1): p. 67-71.

[29] Cushing, B. and C.S. Carter, *Peripheral pulses of oxytocin increase partner preferences in female, but not male, prairie voles.* Horm. Behav., 2000. 37: p. 49-56.

[30] Insel, T.R. and T. Hulihan, *A gender-specific mechanism for pair bonding: Oxytocin and partner preference formation in monogamous voles.* Behav. Neurosci., 1995. 109: p. 782-789.

[31] Veenema, A.H., I.D. Neumann, and L. Rainer, *Central vasopressin and oxytocin release: regulation of complex social behaviours*, in *Progress in Brain Research*. 2008, Elsevier. p. 261-276.

[32] Lonstein, J.S. and S.C. Gammie, *Sensory, hormonal, and neural controls of maternal aggression in laboratory rodents.* Neuroscience and Biobehav. Rev., 2002. 26: p. 869-888.

[33] Consiglio, A.R. and A.B. Lucion, *Lesion of hypothalamic paraventricular nucleus and maternal aggressive behavior in female rats.* Physiology and Behavior, 1996. 59(4): p. 591-596.

[34] Ferris, C.F., K.B. Foote, H.M. Meltser, M.G. Plenby, K.L. Smith, and T.R. Insel, *Oxytocin in the Amygdala Facilitates Maternal Aggression.* Annals of the New York Academy of Sciences, 1992. 652(Oxytocin in Materials, Sexual, and Social Behaviors): p. 456-457.

[35] Consiglio, A.R., A. Borsoi, G.A.M. Pereira, and A.B. Lucion, *Effects of oxytocin microinjected into the central amygdaloid nucleus and bed nucleus of stria terminalis on maternal aggressive behavior in rats.* Physiology & Behavior, 2005. 85(3): p. 354-362.

[36] Bosch, O.J., S.A. Kromer, P.J. Brunton, and I.D. Neumann, *Release of Oxytocin in the hypothalamic paraventricular nucleus, but not central amygdala or lateral septum in lactating residents and virgin intruders during maternal defense.* Neuroscience, 2004. 124: p. 439-448.

[37] Bosch, O.J., S.L. Meddle, D.I. Beiderbeck, A.J. Douglas, and I.D. Neumann, *Brain Oxytocin Correlates with Maternal Aggression: Link to Anxiety.* J. Neurosci., 2005. 25(29): p. 6807-6815.

[38] Veenema, A.H., R. Bredewold, and I.D. Neumann, *Opposite effects of maternal separation on intermale and maternal aggression in C57BL/6 mice: Link to hypothalamic vasopressin and oxytocin immunoreactivity.* Psychoneuroendocrinology, 2007. 32(5): p. 437-450.

[39] Giovenardi, M., M.J. Padoin, L.P. Cadore, and A.B. Lucion, *Hypothalamic paraventricular nucleus, oxytocin, and maternal aggression in rats.* Annals of the New York Academy of Sciences, 1997. 807: p. 606-609.

[40] Lubin, D.A., J.C. Elliot, M.C. Black, and J.M. Johns, *An oxytocin antagonist infused into the central nucleus of the amygdala increases maternal aggressive behavior.* Behav. Neurosci., 2003. 117(2): p. 195-201.

[41] Ragnauth, A.K., N. Devidze, V. Moy, K. Finley, A. Goodwillie, L.M. Kow, L.J. Muglia, and D.W. Pfaff, *Female oxytocin gene-knockout mice, in a semi-natural environment, display exaggerated aggressive behavior.* Genes, Brain & Behavior, 2005. 4(4): p. 229-239.

[42] Elliot, J.C., D.A. Lubin, C.H. Walker, and J.M. Johns, *Acute cocaine alters oxytocin levels in the medial preoptic area and amygdala in lactating rat dams: implications for cocaine-induced changes in maternal behavior and maternal aggression.* Neuropeptides, 2001. 35(2): p. 127-134.

[43] Johns, J.M., C.J. Nelson, K.E. Meter, D.A. Lubin, C.D. Couch, A. Ayers, and C.H. Walker, *Dose-dependent effects of multiple acute cocaine injections on maternal behavior and aggression in Sprague-Dawley rats.* Developmental Neuroscience, 1998. 20(6): p. 525-532.

[44] Johns, J.M., L.R. Noonan, L. Li, and C.A. Pedersen, *Effects of chronic and acute cocaine treatment on the onset of maternal behavior and aggression in Sprague-Dawley rats.* Behav. Neurosci., 1994. 108(1): p. 107-112.

[45] Nephew, B.C., R.S. Bridges, D.F. Lovelock, and E.M. Byrnes, *Enhanced maternal aggression and associated changes in neuropeptide gene expression in reproductively experienced rats.* Behavioral Neuroscience, 2009. 123(5): p. 949-957.

[46] Pedersen, C.A., J.A. Ascher, Y.L. Monroe, and A.J. Prange, *Oxytocin induces maternal behavior in virgin female rats.* Science, 1982. 216(4546): p. 648-650.

[47] Pedersen, C.A. and A.J. Prange Jr., *Induction of maternal behavior in virgin rats after intracerebroventricular administration of oxytocin.* PNAS, 1979. 76: p. 6661-6665.

[48] Bosch, O.J. and I.D. Neumann, *Brain vasopressin is an important regulator of maternal behavior independent of dams' trait anxiety.* PNAS, 2008. 105: p. 17139-17144.

[49] Pedersen, C.A., J.D. Caldwell, C. Walker, G. Ayers, and G.A. Mason, *Oxytocin activates the postpartum onset of rat maternal behavior in the ventral tegmental and preoptic areas.* Behavioral Neuroscience, 1994. 108(6): p. 1163-1171.

[50] van Leengoed, E., E. Kerker, and H.H. Swanson, *Inhibition of post-partum maternal behavior in the rat by injecting an oxytocin antagonist into the cerebral ventricles.* J. Endo., 1987. 112(2): p. 275-282.

[51] Takayanagi, Y., M. Yoshida, I. Bielsky, H. Ross, M. Kawamata, T. Onaka, T. Yanagisawa, T. Kimura, M. Matzuk, L. Young, and K. Nishimori, *Pervasive social deficits, but normal parturition, in oxytocin receptor-deficient mice.* Proc Natl Acad Sci USA, 2005. 102: p. 16096 - 16101.

[52] Kendrick, K.M., *Neural control of maternal behavior and olfactory recognition of offspring.* Brain Res. Bull., 1997. 44: p. 383-395.

[53] DaCosta, A.P.C., R.G. GuevaraGuzman, S. Ohkura, J.A. Goode, and K.M. Kendrick, *The role of oxytocin release in the paraventricular nucleus in the control of maternal behaviour in the sheep.* J Neuroendocrinol, 1996. 8: p. 163-177.

[54] Champagne, F., J. Diorio, S. Sharma, and M.J. Meaney, *Naturally occurring variations in maternal behaivor in the rat are associated with differences in estrogen-inducible central oxytocin receptors.* PNAS, 2001. 98(22): p. 12736-12741.

[55] Francis, D.D., L.J. Young, M.J. Meaney, and T.B. Insel, *Naturally occurring differences in maternal care are associated with the expression of oxytocin and vasopressin (V1a) receptors: Gender differences.* J. Neuroendocrinology, 2002. 14: p. 349-353.

[56] Shahrokh, D.K., T.-Y. Zhang, J. Diorio, A. Gratton, and M.J. Meaney, *Oxytocin-Dopamine Interactions Mediate Variations in Maternal Behavior in the Rat.* Endocrinology, 2010. 151(5): p. 2276-2286.

[57] Champagne, F.A. and M.J. Meaney, *Stress During Gestation Alters Postpartum Maternal Care and the Development of the Offspring in a Rodent Model.* Biological Psychiatry, 2006. 59(12): p. 1227-1235.

[58] Olazabal, D.E. and L.J. Young, *Oxytocin receptors in the nucleus accumbens facilitate /`spontaneous/' maternal behavior in female prairie voles.* Hormones Behav, 2005. 48: p. 177.

[59] Neumann, I.D., L. Torner, and A. Wigger, *Brain oxytocin: differential inhibition of neuroendocrine stress responses and anxiety-related behaviour in virgin, pregnant and lactating rats.* Neuroscience, 2000. 95: p. 567-575.

[60] McCarthy, M.M., C.H. McDonald, P.J. Brooks, and D. Goldman, *An anxiolytic action of oxytocin is enhanced by estrogen in the mouse.* Physiol Behav, 1996. 60: p. 1209-1215.

[61] Caughey, S.D., S.M. Klampfl, V.R. Bishop, J. Pfoertsch, I.D. Neumann, O.J. Bosch, and S.L. Meddle, *Changes in the Intensity of Maternal Aggression and Central Oxytocin and Vasopressin V1a Receptors Across the Peripartum Period in the Rat.* Journal of Neuroendocrinology, 2011. 23(11): p. 1113-1124.

[62] Windle, R.J., N. Shanks, S.L. Lightman, and C.D. Ingram, *Central oxytocin administration reduces stress-induced corticosterone release and anxiety behavior in rats.* Endocrinology, 1997. 138: p. 2829-2834.

[63] Piccinelli, M. and G. Wilkinson, *Gender differences in depression.* The British Journal of Psychiatry, 2000. 177(6): p. 486-492.

[64] Engelmann, M., K. Ebner, C.T. Wotjak, and R. Landgraf, *Endogenous oxytocin is involved in short-term olfactory memory in female rats.* Behavioral Brain Res., 1998. 90: p. 89-94.

[65] Lee, H.-J., H.K. Caldwell, A.H. Macbeth, and W.S. Young Iii, *Behavioural studies using temporal and spatial inactivation of the oxytocin receptor*, in *Progress in Brain Research*, D.N. Inga and L. Rainer, Editors. 2008, Elsevier. p. 73-77.

[66] Lévy, F., K.M. Kendrick, J.A. Goode, R. Guevara-Guzman, and E.B. Keverne, *Oxytocin and vasopressin release in the olfactory bulb of parturient ewes: changes with maternal experience and effects on acetylcholine, γ-aminobutyric acid, glutamate and noradrenaline release.* Brain Research, 1995. 669(2): p. 197-206.

[67] Campbell, A., *Attachment, aggression and affiliation: The role of oxytocin in female social behavior.* Biological Psychology, 2008. 77(1): p. 1-10.

[68] Nephew, B.C. and R.S. Bridges, *Arginine vasopressin V1a receptor antagonist impairs maternal memory in rats.* Physiology & Behavior, 2008. 95(1-2): p. 182-186.

[69] Byrnes, E.M. and R.S. Bridges, *Endogenous opioid facilitation of maternal memory in rats.* Behavioral Neuroscience, 2000. 114(4): p. 797-804.

[70] D'Cunha, T.M., S.J. King, A.S. Fleming, and F. Lévy, *Oxytocin receptors in the nucleus accumbens shell are involved in the consolidation of maternal memory in postpartum rats.* Hormones and Behavior, 2011. 59(1): p. 14-21.

[71] Kendrick, K.M., *Oxytocin, motherhood and bonding.* Experimental Physiology, 2000. 85: p. 111s-124s.

[72] Kosfeld, M., M. Heinrichs, P.J. Zak, U. Fischbacher, and E. Fehr, *Oxytocin increases trust in humans.* Nature, 2005. 435: p. 673-676.

[73] Zak, P.J., R. Kurzban, and W.T. Matzner, *Oxytocin is associated with human trustworthiness.* Hormones and Behavior, 2005. 48(5): p. 522-527.

[74] Rilling, J.K., A.C. DeMarco, P.D. Hackett, R. Thompson, B. Ditzen, R. Patel, and G. Pagnoni, *Effects of intranasal oxytocin and vasopressin on cooperative behavior and associated brain activity in men.* Psychoneuroendocrinology, 2012. 37(4): p. 447-461.

[75] Grewen, K.M., S.S. Girdler, J. Amico, and K.C. Light, *Effects of Partner Support on Resting Oxytocin, Cortisol, Norepinephrine, and Blood Pressure Before and After Warm Partner Contact.* Psychosomatic Medicine, 2005. 67(4): p. 531-538.

[76] Carmichael, M.S., *Plasma oxytocin increases in the human sexual response.* J. Clin. Endocrinol. Metab., 1987. 64: p. 27-31.

[77] Murphy, M.R., J.R. Seckl, S. Burton, S.A. Checkley, and S.L. Lightman, *Changes in oxytocin and vasopressin secretion during sexual activity in men.* J. Clin. Endocrinol. Metab., 1987. 65: p. 738-741.

[78] Kruger, T., P. Haake, D. Chereath, W. Knapp, O. Janssen, M. Exton, M. Schedlowski, and U. Hartmann, *Specificity of the neuroendocrine response to orgasm during sexual arousal in men.* Journal of Endocrinology, 2003. 177(1): p. 57-64.

[79] Modahl, C., L.A. Green, D. Fein, M. Morris, L. Waterhouse, C. Feinstein, and H. Levin, *Plasma oxytocin levels in autistic children.* Biological Psychiatry, 1998. 43(4): p. 270-277.

[80] Gregory, S., J. Connelly, A. Towers, J. Johnson, D. Biscocho, C. Markunas, C. Lintas, R. Abramson, H. Wright, P. Ellis, C. Langford, G. Worley, G.R. Delong, S. Murphy, M. Cuccaro, A. Persico, and M. Pericak-Vance, *Genomic and epigenetic evidence for oxytocin receptor deficiency in autism.* BMC Medicine, 2009. 7(1): p. 62.

[81] Sebat, J., B. Lakshmi, D. Malhotra, J. Troge, C. Lese-Martin, T. Walsh, B. Yamrom, S. Yoon, A. Krasnitz, J. Kendall, A. Leotta, D. Pai, R. Zhang, Y. Lee, J. Hicks, S. Spence, A. Lee, K. Puura, T. Lehtimaki, D. Ledbetter, P. Gregersen, J. Bregman, J. Sutcliffe, V. Jobanputra, W. Chung, D. Warburton, M. King, D. Skuse, D. Geschwind, and T. Gilliam, *Strong association of de novo copy number mutations with autism.* Science, 2007. 316: p. 445 - 449.

[82] Andari, E., J.-R. Duhamel, T. Zalla, E. Herbrecht, M. Leboyer, and A. Sirigu, *Promoting social behavior with oxytocin in high-functioning autism spectrum disorders.* Proceedings of the National Academy of Sciences, 2010. 107(9): p. 4389-4394.

[83] Hollander, E., S. Novotny, M. Hanratty, R. Yaffe, C.M. DeCaria, B.R. Aronowitz, and S. Mosovich, *Oxytocin Infusion Reduces Repetitive Behaviors in Adults with Autistic and Asperger's Disorders.* Neuropsychopharmacology, 2002. 28(1): p. 193-198.

[84] Guastella, A.J., S.L. Einfeld, K.M. Gray, N.J. Rinehart, B.J. Tonge, T.J. Lambert, and I.B. Hickie, *Intranasal Oxytocin Improves Emotion Recognition for Youth with Autism Spectrum Disorders.* Biological Psychiatry, 2010. 67(7): p. 692-694.

[85] Guastella, A.J., A.L. Howard, M.R. Dadds, P. Mitchell, and D.S. Carson, *A randomized controlled trial of intranasal oxytocin as an adjunct to exposure therapy for social anxiety disorder.* Psychoneuroendocrinology, 2009. 34(6): p. 917-923.

[86] Feldman, R., I. Gordon, I. Schneiderman, O. Weisman, and O. Zagoory-Sharon, *Natural variations in maternal and paternal care are associated with systematic changes in oxytocin following parent–infant contact.* Psychoneuroendocrinology, 2010. 35(8): p. 1133-1141.

[87] Naber, F., M.H. van Ijzendoorn, P. Deschamps, H. van Engeland, and M.J. Bakermans-Kranenburg, *Intranasal oxytocin increases fathers' observed responsiveness during play with their children: A double-blind within-subject experiment.* Psychoneuroendocrinology, 2010. 35(10): p. 1583-1586.

[88] Gordon, I., O. Zagoory-Sharon, J.F. Leckman, and R. Feldman, *Oxytocin, cortisol, and triadic family interactions.* Physiology and Behavior, 2010. 101(5): p. 679-684.

[89] Gordon, I., O. Zagoory-Sharon, J.F. Leckman, and R. Feldman, *Oxytocin and the development of parenting in humans.* Biol Psychiatry, 2010. 68: p. 377-382.

[90] Keverne, E.B. and J.P. Curley, *Vasopressin, oxytocin, and social behavior.* Curr. Opin. Neurobiol., 2004. 14: p. 777-783.

[91] Insel, T.R., *The challenge of translation in social neuroscience: a review of oxytocin, vasopressin, and affiliative behavior.* Neuron, 2010. 65: p. 768-779.

[92] Frasch, A., T. Zetzsche, A. Steiger, and G.F. Jirikowski, *Reduction of plasma oxytocin levels in patients suffering from major depression.* Adv Exp Med Biol, 1995. 395: p. 257-258.

[93] Zetzsche, T., A. Frasch, G. Jirikowski, H. Murck, and A. Steiger, *Nocturnal oxytocin secretion is reduced in major depression.* Biological Psychiatry, 1996. 39(7): p. 584-584.

[94] Scantamburlo, G., M. Hansenne, S. Fuchs, W. Pitchot, P. Marechal, and C. Pequeux, *Plasma oxytocin levels and anxiety in patients with major depression.* Psychoneuroendocrinology, 2007. 32: p. 407-410.

[95] Van Londen, L., J.G. Goekoop, G.M. van Kempen, A.C. Frankhuijzen-Sierevogel, V.M. Wiegant, E.A. van der Velde, and D. De Wied, *Plasma levels of arginine vasopressin elevated in patients with major depression.* Neuropsychopharmacology, 1997. 17: p. 284-292.

[96] Purba, J.S., W.J.G. Hoogendijk, M.A. Hofman, and D.F. Swaab, *Increased Number of Vasopressin- and Oxytocin-Expressing Neurons in the Paraventricular Nucleus of the Hypothalamus in Depression.* Arch Gen Psychiatry, 1996. 53(2): p. 137-143.

[97] Meynen, G., U.A. Unmehopa, M.A. Hofman, D.F. Swaab, and W.J.G. Hoogendijk, *Hypothalamic oxytocin mRNA expression and melancholic depression.* Mol Psychiatry, 2007. 12(2): p. 118-119.

[98] Hurlemann, R., A. Patin, O.A. Onur, M.X. Cohen, T. Baumgartner, S. Metzler, I. Dziobek, J. Gallinat, M. Wagner, W. Maier, and K.M. Kendrick, *Oxytocin Enhances Amygdala-Dependent, Socially Reinforced Learning and Emotional Empathy in Humans.* The Journal of Neuroscience, 2010. 30(14): p. 4999-5007.

[99] Evans, S., S.S. Shergill, and B.B. Averbeck, *Oxytocin Decreases Aversion to Angry Faces in an Associative Learning Task.* Neuropsychopharmacology, 2010. 35(13): p. 2502-2509.

[100] Pedersen, C.A., *Biological Aspects of Social Bonding and the Roots of Human Violence.* Annals of the New York Academy of Sciences, 2004. 1036(1): p. 106-127.

[101] Ditzen, B., M. Schaer, B. Gabriel, G. Bodenmann, U. Ehlert, and M. Heinrichs, *Intranasal Oxytocin Increases Positive Communication and Reduces Cortisol Levels During Couple Conflict.* Biological Psychiatry, 2009. 65(9): p. 728-731.

[102] Taylor, S.E., *Tend and befriend.* Curr Dir Psychol Sci, 2006. 15: p. 273-277.

[103] Turner, R.A., M. Altemus, T. Enos, B. Cooper, and T. McGuinness, *Preliminary research on plasma oxytocin in normal cycling women: Investigating emotion and interpersonal distress.* Psychiatry: Interpersonal and Biological Processes, 1999. 62(2): p. 97-113.

[104] Turner, R.A., M. Altemus, D.N. Yip, E. Kupferman, D. Fletcher, A. Bostrom, D.M. Lyons, and J.A. Amico, *Effects of Emotion on Oxytocin, Prolactin, and ACTH in Women.* Stress, 2002. 5(4): p. 269-276.

[105] Taylor, S.E., S. Saphire-Bernstein, and T.E. Seeman, *Are Plasma Oxytocin in Women and Plasma Vasopressin in Men Biomarkers of Distressed Pair-Bond Relationships?* Psychological Science, 2010. 21(1): p. 3-7.

[106] Nelson, E.E. and J. Panksepp, *Brain substrates of infant-mother attachment: Contributions of opioids, oxytocin, and norepinephrine.* Neurosci Biobehav Rev, 1998. 22: p. 437-452.

[107] Levine, A., O. Zagoory-Sharon, R. Feldman, and A. Weller, *Oxytocin during pregnancy and early postpartum: Individual patterns and maternal-fetal attachment.* Peptides, 2007. 28: p. 1162-1169.

[108] Feldman, R., A. Weller, O. Zagoory-Sharon, and A. Levine, *Evidence for a neuroendocrinological foundation of human affiliation: plasma oxytocin levels across pregnancy and the postpartum period predict mother-infant bonding.* Psychol Sci, 2007. 18: p. 965-970.

[109] Broad, K.D., J.P. Curley, and E.B. Keverne, *Mother–infant bonding and the evolution of mammalian social relationships.* Philosophical Transactions of the Royal Society B: Biological Sciences, 2006. 361(1476): p. 2199-2214.

[110] Bartels, A. and S. Zeki, *The neural correlates of maternal and romantic love.* Neuroimage, 2004. 21: p. 1155-1166.

[111] Uvnäs-Mobcrg, K., A.-M. Widström, E. Nissen, and H. Björvell, *Personality traits in women 4 days postpartum and their correlation with plasma levels of oxytocin and prolactin.* Journal of Psychosomatic Obstetrics & Gynecology, 1990. 11(4): p. 261-273.

[112] Bakermans-Kranenburg, M.J. and M.H. van IJzendoorn, *Oxytocin receptor (OXTR) and serotonin transporter (5-HTT) genes associated with observed parenting.* Social Cognitive and Affective Neuroscience, 2008. 3(2): p. 128-134.

[113] Bakermans-Kranenburg, M.J., M.H. van Ijzendoorn, M.M.E. Riem, M. Tops, and L.R.A. Alink, *Oxytocin decreases handgrip force in reaction to infant crying in females without harsh parenting experiences.* Social Cognitive and Affective Neuroscience, 2011.

[114] Light, K.C., K.M. Grewen, J.A. Amico, M. Boccia, K.A. Brownley, and J.M. Johns, *Deficits in plasma oxytocin responses and increased negative affect, stress, and blood pressure in mothers with cocaine exposure during pregnancy.* Addictive Behaviors, 2004. 29(8): p. 1541-1564.

[115] Strathearn, L., P. Fonagy, J. Amico, and P.R. Montague, *Adult attachment predicts maternal brain and oxytocin response to infant cues.* Neuropsychopharm, 2009. 34: p. 2655-2666.

[116] Skrundz, M., M. Bolten, I. Nast, D.H. Hellhammer, and G. Meinlschmidt, *Plasma Oxytocin Concentration during Pregnancy is associated with Development of Postpartum Depression.* Neuropsychopharmacology, 2011. 36(9): p. 1886-1893.

[117] Ozsoy, S., E. Esel, and M. Kula, *Serum oxytocin levels in patients with depression and the effects of gender and antidepressant treatment.* Psychiatry Res, 2009. 169: p. 249-252.

[118] Cyranowski, J.M., T.L. Hofkens, E. Frank, H. Seltman, H.-M. Cai, and J.A. Amico, *Evidence of Dysregulated Peripheral Oxytocin Release Among Depressed Women.* Psychosomatic Medicine, 2008. 70(9): p. 967-975.

[119] Heim, C. and E.B. Binder, *Current research trends in early life stress and depression: Review of human studies on sensitive periods, gene–environment interactions, and epigenetics.* Experimental Neurology, 2011. 233(1): p. 102-111.

[120] Heim, C., L.J. Young, D.J. Newport, T. Mletzko, A.H. Miller, and C.B. Nemeroff, *Lower CSF oxytocin concentrations in women with a history of childhood abuse.* Mol Psychiatry, 2008. 14(10): p. 954-958.

[121] Steube, A.M., K.M. Grewen, C.A. Pedersen, C. Propper, and S. Meltzer-Brody, *Failed actation and perinatal depression: Common problems with shared neuroendocrine mechanism.* J. Women's Health, 2011. 21(3): p. 264-272.

[122] Onaka, T., Y. Takayanagi, and M. Yoshida, *Roles of Oxytocin Neurones in the Control of Stress, Energy Metabolism, and Social Behaviour.* Journal of Neuroendocrinology, 2012. 24(4): p. 587-598.

[123] Rimmele, U., K. Hediger, M. Heinrichs, and P. Klaver, *Oxytocin makes a face in memory amiliar.* J Neurosci, 2009. 29: p. 38-42.

[124] Wang, Z., C.F. Ferris, and G.J.D. Vries, *Role of Septal Vasopressin Innervation in Paternal Behavior in Prairie Voles (Microtus ochrogaster).* Proceedings of the National Academy of Sciences, 1994. 91(1): p. 400-404.

[125] Winslow, J., N. Hastings, C.S. Carter, C. Harbaugh, and T.R. Insel, *A role for central vasopressin in pair bonding in monogamous prairie voles.* Nature, 1993. 365: p. 545-548.

[126] Pitkow, L.J., *Facilitation of affiliation and pair-bond formation by vasopressin receptor gene transfer into the ventral forebrain of a monogamous vole.* J. Neurosci., 2001. 21: p. 7392-7396.

[127] Lim, M.M., *Enhanced partner preference in promiscuous species by manipulating the expression of a single gene.* Nature, 2004. 429: p. 754-757.

[128] Lim, M.M. and L.J. Young, *Vasopressin-dependent neural circuits underlying pair bond ormation in the monogamous prairie vole.* Neuroscience, 2004. 125: p. 35-45.

[129] Goodson, J.L. and A.H. Bass, *Social behavior functions and related anatomical characteristics of vasotocin/vasopressin systems in vertebrates.* Brain Res. Rev., 2001. 35: p. 246-265.

[130] Ferris, C.F., D.M. Meenan, J.F. Axelson, and H.E. Albers, *A vasopressin antagonist can reverse dominant/subordinate behavior in hamsters.* Physiology and Behavior, 1986. 38: p. 135-138.

[131] Ferris, C.F. and M. Potegal, *Vasopressin receptor blockade in the anterior hypothalamus suppresses aggression in hamsters.* Physiol. and Behav., 1988. 44: p. 235-239.

[132] Bester-Meredith, J.K., P.A. Martin, and C.A. Marler, *Manipulations of Vasopressin alter aggression differently across testing conditions in monogamous and non-monogamous Peromyscus mice.* Aggressive Behavior, 2005. 31: p. 189-199.

[133] Caldwell, H.K. and H.E. Albers, *Effect of photoperiod on vasopressin induced aggression in Syrian hamsters.* Horm. and Behav., 2004. 46: p. 444-449.

[134] Gobrogge, K.L., Y. Liu, L.J. Young, and Z. Wang, *Anterior hypothalamic vasopressin regulates pair-bonding and drug-induced aggression in a monogamous rodent.* Proceedings of the National Academy of Sciences, 2009. 106(45): p. 19144-19149.

[135] Ferris, C.F., R.H. Melloni, G. Koppel, K.W. Perry, R.W. Fuller, and Y. Delville, *Vasopressin/serotonin interactions in the anterior hypothalamus control aggressive behavior in golden hamsters.* J Neurosci, 1997. 17: p. 4331 - 4340.

[136] Albers, E.H., A. Dean, M.C. Karom, D. Smith, and K.L. Huhman, *Role of V1a vasopressin receptors in the control of aggression in Syrian hamsters.* Brain Research, 2006. 1073-1074: p. 425-430.

[137] Ferris, C.F., S. Lu, T. Messenger, C.D. Guillon, N. Heindel, M. Miller, G. Koppel, F.R. Bruns, and N.G. Simon, *Orally active vasopressin V1a receptor antagonist, SRX251, selectively blocks aggressive behavior.* Pharm. Biochem. Behav., 2006. 83: p. 169-174.

[138] Melloni Jr, R.H. and L.A. Ricci, *Adolescent exposure to anabolic/androgenic steroids and the neurobiology of offensive aggression: A hypothalamic neural model based on findings in pubertal Syrian hamsters.* Hormones and Behavior, 2010. 58(1): p. 177-191.

[139] Carter, C.S., E.M. Boone, H. Pounajafi-Nazarloo, and K.L. Bales, *Consequences of early experiences and exposure to oxytocin and vasopressin are sexuallly dimorphic.* Developmental Neurosci., 2009. 31(4): p. 25-37.

[140] Parker, K.J. and T.M. Lee, *Central vasopressin administration regulates the onset of acultative paternal behavior in Microtus pennsylvanicus (Meadow voles).* Horm. Behav., 2001. 39: p. 285-294.

[141] Bester-Meredith, J.K., L.J. Young, and C.A. Marler, *Species differences in paternal behavior and aggression in Peromyscus and their associations with vasopressin immunoreactivity and receptors.* Hormones and Behavior, 1999. 36: p. 25-38.

[142] Bester-Meredith, J.K. and C.A. Marler, *The Association between male offspring aggression and paternal and maternal behavior of Peromyscus mice.* Ethology, 2003. 109(10): p. 797-808.

[143] Liebsch, G., C.T. Wotjak, R. Landgraf, and M. Engelmann, *Septal vasopressin modulates anxiety-related behaviour in rats.* Neurosci Lett, 1996. 217: p. 101-104.

[144] Englemann, M., C.T. Wotjak, K. Ebner, and R. Landgraf, *Behavioural impact of ntraseptally released vasopressin and oxytocin in rats.* Experimental Physiology, 2000. 85: p. 125s-130s.

[145] Appenrodt, E., R. Schnabel, and H. Schwarzberg, *Vasopressin administration modulates anxiety-related behavior in rats.* Physiology & Behavior, 1998. 64(4): p. 543-547.

[146] Egashira, N., A. Tanoue, T. Matsuda, E. Koushi, S. Harada, Y. Takano, G. Tsujimoto, K. Mishima, K. Iwasaki, and M. Fujiwara, *Impaired social interaction and reduced anxiety-related behavior in vasopressin V1a receptor knockout mice.* Behavioural Brain Research, 2007. 178(1): p. 123-127.

[147] Caldwell, H. and W. Young, *Oxytocin and vasopressin: genetics and behavioral implications.* Handbook of Neurochemistry and Molecular Neurobiology Neuroactive Proteins and Peptides, 2006(3): p. 573-607.

[148] Griebel, G., J. Simiand, C.S.L. Gal, J. Wagnon, M. Pascal, and B. Scatton, *Anxiolytic- and antidepressant-like effects of the non-peptide vasopressin V-1b receptor antagonist, SSR149415, suggest an innovative approach for the treatment of stress-related disorders.* Proc Natl Acad Sci USA, 2002. 99: p. 6370-6375.

[149] Serradeil-Le Gal, C., J. Wagnon, J. Simiand, G. Griebel, C. Lacour, and G. Guillon, *Characterization of (2S,4R)-1-[lsqb]5-chloro-1-[lsqb](2,4-dimethoxyphenyl)sulfonyl[rsqb]-3-(2-methoxy-phenyl)-2-oxo-2,3-dihydro-1H-indol-3-yl[rsqb]-4-hydroxy-N,N-dimethyl-2-pyrrolidine carboxamide (SSR149415), a selective and orally active vasopressin V1b receptor antagonist.* J Pharmacol Exp Ther, 2002. 300: p. 1122-1130.

[150] Serradeil-Le, G.C., S. Derick, G. Brossard, M. Manning, J. Simiand, and R. Gaillard, *Functional and pharmacological characterization of the first specific agonist and antagonist for the V1b receptor in mammals.* Stress, 2003. 6: p. 199-206.

[151] Wersinger, S.R., E.I. Ginnns, A.M. O'Carroll, S.J. Lolait, and W.S. Young Iii, *Vasopressin V1b receptor knockout reduces aggressive behavior in male mice.* Molecular Psychiatry, 2002. 7(9): p. 975-984.

[152] Bosch, O.J., S.A. Kromer, and I.D. Neumann, *Prenatal stress: opposite effects on anxiety and hypothalamic expression of vasopressin and corticotropin releasing hormone in rats selectively bred for high and low anxiety.* Eur. J. Neurosci., 2006. 23: p. 541-551.

[153] Keck, M.E., A. Wigger, T. Welt, M.B. Muller, A. Gesing, and J. Reul, *Vasopressin mediates the response of the combined dexamethasone//CRH test in hyper-anxious rats: implications for pathogenesis of affective disorders.* Neuropsychopharmacology, 2002. 26: p. 94-105.

[154] Wigger, A., M.M. Sanchez, K.C. Mathys, K. Ebner, E. Frank, and D. Liu, *Alterations in central neuropeptide expression, release, and receptor binding in rats bred for high anxiety: critical role of vasopressin.* Neuropsychopharmacology, 2004. 29: p. 1-14.

[155] Landgraf, R., M.S. Keler, M. Bunck, C. Murgatroyd, D. Spengler, M. Zimbelmann, M. Nubaumer, L. Czibere, C.W. Turck, N. Singewald, D. Rujescu, and E. Frank, *Candidate genes of anxiety-related behavior in HAB/LAB rats and mice: Focus on vasopressin and glyoxalase-I.* Neuroscience & Biobehavioral Reviews, 2007. 31(1): p. 89-102.

[156] Murgatroyd, C., A. Wigger, E. Frank, N. Singewald, M. Bunck, F. Holsboer, R. Landgraf, and D. Spengler, *Impaired repression at a vasopressin promoter polymorphism underlies overexpression of vasopressin in a rat model of trait anxiety.* J. Neurosci., 2004. 24(35): p. 7762-7770.

[157] Porsolt, R., M. Le Pichon, and M. Jalfre, *Depression: a new animal model sensitive to antidepressant treatments.* Nature, 1977. 266: p. 730-732.

[158] Wotjak, C.T., J. Ganster, G. Kohl, F. Holsboer, R. Landgraf, and M. Engelmann, *Dissociated central and peripheral release of vasopressin, but not oxytocin, in response to repeated swim stress: New insights into the secretory capacities of peptidergic neurons.* Neuroscience, 1998. 85: p. 1209-1222.

[159] Ebner, K., C.T. Wotjak, F. Holsboer, R. Landgraf, and M. Engelmann, *Vasopressin released within the septal brain area during swim stress modulates the behavioral stress response in rats.* Eur J Neurosci, 1999. 11: p. 997-1002.

[160] Ebner, K., C.T. Wotjak, R. Landgraf, and M. Engelmann, *Forced swimming triggers vasopressin release within the amygdala to modulate stress-coping strategies in rats.* Eur J Neurosci, 2002. 15: p. 384-388.

[161] Salomé, N., J. Stemmelin, C. Cohen, and G. Griebel, *Differential roles of amygdaloid nuclei n the anxiolytic- and antidepressant-like effects of the V1b receptor antagonist, SSR149415, in rats.* Psychopharmacology, 2006. 187(2): p. 237-244.

[162] Engelmann, M., M. Ludwig, and R. Landgraf, *Simultaneous monitoring of intracerebral release and behavior: vasopressin improves social recognition.* J Neuroendocrinol, 1994. 6: p. 391-395.

[163] Landgraf, R., R. Gerstberger, A. Montkowski, J.C. Probst, C.T. Wotjak, and F. Holsboer, *V1 vasopressin receptor antisense oligodeoxynucleotide into septum reduces vasopressin binding, social discrimination abilities, and anxiety-related behavior in rats.* J Neurosci, 1995. 15: p. 4250-4258.

[164] Landgraf, R., E. Frank, J.M. Aldag, I.D. Neumann, X. Ren, and E.F. Terwilliger, *Viral vector-mediated gene transfer of the vole V1a vasopressin receptor in the rat septum: improved social discrimination and active social behavior.* J Neuroendocrinol, 2003. 18: p. 403-411.

[165] Wersinger, S.R., H.K. Caldwell, L. Martinez, P. Gold, S.B. Hu, and W.S. Young, *Vasopressin 1a receptor knockout mice have a subtle olfactory deficit but normal aggression.* Genes, Brain and Behavior, 2007. 6(6): p. 540-551.

[166] Aarde, S.M. and J.D. Jentsch, *Haploinsufficiency of the arginine–vasopressin gene is associated with poor spatial working memory performance in rats.* Hormones and Behavior, 2006. 49(4): p. 501-508.

[167] Alescio-Lautier, B., V. Paban, and B. Soumireu-Mourat, *Neuromodulation of memory in the hippocampus by vasopressin.* European Journal of Pharmacology, 2000. 405(1–3): p. 63-72.

[168] Gaffori, O.J.W. and D. De Wied, *Time-related memory effects of vasopressin analogues in rats.* Pharmacology Biochemistry and Behavior, 1986. 25(6): p. 1125-1129.

[169] Young, L.J. and Z. Wang, *The neurobiology of pair bonding.* Nature Neurosci., 2004. 7(10): p. 1048-1054.

[170] Cho, M.M., A.C. DeVries, J.R. Williams, and C.S. Carter, *The effects of oxytocin and vasopressin on partner preferences in male and female prairie voles (Microtus ochrogaster).* Behav. Neurosci., 1999. 113: p. 1071-1079.

[171] Nephew, B.C. and R.S. Bridges, *Central actions of arginine vasopressin and a V1a receptor antagonist on maternal aggression, maternal behavior, and grooming in lactating rats.* Pharmacology Biochemistry and Behavior, 2008. 91(1): p. 77-83.

[172] Nephew, B.C., E.M. Byrnes, and R.S. Bridges, *Vasopressin mediates enhanced offspring protection in multiparous rats.* Neuropharmacology, 2010. 58(1): p. 102-106.

[173] Gutzler, S.J., M. Karom, W.D. Erwin, and H.E. Albers, *Arginine-vasopressin and the regulation of aggression in female Syrian hamsters (Mesocricetus auratus).* European Journal of Neuroscience, 2010. 31(9): p. 1655-1663.

[174] Caffrey, M.K., B.C. Nephew, and M. Febo, *Central vasopressin V1a receptors modulate neural processing in mothers facing intruder threat to pups.* Neuropharmacology, 2010. 58(1): p. 107-116.

[175] Bosch, O.J. and I.D. Neumann, *Vasopressin released within the central amygdala promotes maternal aggression.* European Journal of Neuroscience, 2010. 31(5): p. 883-891.

[176] Kessler, M.S., O.J. Bosch, M. Bunck, R. Landgraf, and I.D. Neumann, *Maternal care differs n mice bred for high vs. low trait anxiety: Impact of brain vasopressin and cross-fostering.* Social Neuroscience, 2010. 6(2): p. 156-168.

[177] Curley, J.P., C.L. Jensen, B. Franks, and F.A. Champagne, *Variation in maternal and anxiety-like behavior associated with discrete patterns of oxytocin and vasopressin 1a receptor density in the lateral septum.* Hormones and Behavior, 2012. 61(3): p. 454-461.

[178] Wersinger, S.R., J.L. Temple, H.K. Caldwell, and W.S. Young, *Inactivation of the Oxytocin and the Vasopressin (Avp) 1b Receptor Genes, But Not the Avp 1a Receptor Gene, Differentially Impairs the Bruce Effect in Laboratory Mice (Mus musculus).* Endocrinology, 2008. 149(1): p. 116-121.

[179] Guastella, A.J., A.R. Kenyon, G.A. Alvares, D.S. Carson, and I.B. Hickie, *Intranasal Arginine Vasopressin Enhances the Encoding of Happy and Angry Faces in Humans.* Biological Psychiatry, 2010. 67(12): p. 1220-1222.

[180] Guastella, A.J., A.R. Kenyon, C. Unkelbach, G.A. Alvares, and I.B. Hickie, *Arginine Vasopressin selectively enhances recognition of sexual cues in male humans.* Psychoneuroendocrinology, 2011. 36(2): p. 294-297.

[181] Thompson, R.R., K. George, J.C. Walton, S.P. Orr, and J. Benson, *Sex-specific influences of vasopressin on human social communication.* PNAS, 2006. 103(20): p. 7889-7894.

[182] Thompson, R., S. Gupta, K. Miller, S. Mills, and S. Orr, *The effects of vasopressin on human acial responses related to social communication.* Psychoneuroendocrinology, 2004. 29(1): p. 35-48.

[183] Coccaro, E.F., R.J. Kavoussi, R.L. Hauger, T.B. Cooper, and C.F. Ferris, *Cerebrospinal Fluid Vasopressin Levels: Correlates With Aggression and Serotonin Function in Personality-Disordered Subjects.* Arch Gen Psychiatry, 1998. 55(8): p. 708-714.

[184] Virkkunen, M., R. Rawlings, R. Tokola, R.E. Poland, A. Guidotti, C. Nemeroff, G. Bissette, K. Kalogeras, S.-L. Karonen, and M. Linnoila, *CSF Biochemistries, Glucose Metabolism, and Diurnal Activity Rhythms in Alcoholic, Violent Offenders, Fire Setters, and Healthy Volunteers.* Arch Gen Psychiatry, 1994. 51(1): p. 20-27.

[185] de Kloet, C.S., E. Vermetten, E. Geuze, V.M. Wiegant, and H.G.M. Westenberg, *Elevated plasma arginine vasopressin levels in veterans with posttraumatic stress disorder.* Journal of Psychiatric Research, 2008. 42(3): p. 192-198.

[186] Pitman, R.K., S.P. Orr, and N.B. Lasko, *Effects of intranasal vasopressin and oxytocin on physiologic responding during personal combat imagery in Vietnam veterans with posttraumatic stress disorder.* Psychiatry Research, 1993. 48(2): p. 107-117.

[187] Yehuda, R., J. Flory, L. Pratchett, J. Buxbaum, M. Ising, and F. Holsboer, *Putative biological mechanisms for the association between early life adversity and the subsequent development of PTSD.* Psychopharmacology, 2010. 212(3): p. 405-417.

[188] Gold, P., F. Goodwin, and V. Reus, *Vasopressin in affective illness.* The Lancet, 1978. 311(8076): p. 1233-1236.

[189] Inder, W.J., R.A. Donald, T.C. Prickett, C.M. Frampton, P.F. Sullivan, R.T. Mulder, and P.R. Joyce, *Arginine vasopressin is associated with hypercortisolemia and suicide attempts in depression.* Biol Psychiatry, 1997. 42: p. 744-747.

[190] Merali, Z., P. Kent, L. Du, P. Hrdina, M. Palkovits, G. Faludi, M.O. Poulter, T. Bédard, and H. Anisman, *Corticotropin-Releasing Hormone, Arginine Vasopressin, Gastrin-Releasing Peptide, and Neuromedin B Alterations in Stress-Relevant Brain Regions of Suicides and Control Subjects.* Biological Psychiatry, 2006. 59(7): p. 594-602.

[191] Goekoop, J.G., R. de Winter, R. Wolterbeek, and V. Wiegant, *Support for two increased vasopressinergic activities in depression at large and the differential effect of antidepressant treatment.* Journal of Psychopharmacology, 2010. 25(10): p. 1304-1312.

[192] Goekoop, J.G., R.P.F. de Winter, R. de Rijk, K.H. Zwinderman, A. Frankhuijzen-Sierevogel, and V.M. Wiegant, *Depression with above-normal plasma vasopressin: Validation by relations with family history of depression and mixed anxiety and retardation.* Psychiatry Research, 2006. 141(2): p. 201-211.

[193] van West, D., J. Del-Favero, Y. Aulchenko, P. Oswald, D. Souery, T. Forsgren, S. Sluijs, S. Bel-Kacem, R. Adolfsson, J. Mendlewicz, C. Van Duijn, D. Deboutte, C. Van Broeckhoven, and S. Claes, *A major SNP haplotype of the arginine vasopressin 1B receptor protects against recurrent major depression.* Mol Psychiatry, 2004. 9(3): p. 287-292.

[194] Manning, M., A. Misicka, A. Olma, K. Bankowski, S. Stoev, B. Chini, T. Durroux, B. Mouillac, M. Corbani, and G. Guillon, *Oxytocin and Vasopressin Agonists and Antagonists as Research Tools and Potential Therapeutics.* Journal of Neuroendocrinology, 2012. 24(4): p. 609-628.

[195] Manning, M., S. Stoev, B. Chini, T. Durroux, B. Mouillac, G. Guillon, D.N. Inga, and L. Rainer, *Peptide and non-peptide agonists and antagonists for the vasopressin and oxytocin V1a, V1b, V2 and OT receptors: research tools and potential therapeutic agents*, in *Progress in Brain Research*. 2008, Elsevier. p. 473-512.

[196] Beckwith, B.E., T.V. Petros, P.J. Bergloff, and R.J. Staebler, *Vasopressin analogue (ddavp) acilitates recall of narrative prose.* Behavioral Neuroscience, 1987. 101(3): p. 429-432.

[197] Pietrowsky, R., G. Fehm-Wolfsdorf, J. Born, and H.L. Fehm, *Effects of DGAVP on verbal memory.* Peptides, 1988. 9(6): p. 1361-1366.

[198] Beckwith, B.E., D.I. Couk, and T.S. Till, *Vasopressin analog influences the performance of males on a reaction time task.* Peptides, 1983. 4(5): p. 707-709.

[199] Perras, B., C. Droste, J. Born, H.L. Fehm, and R. Pietrowsky, *Verbal memory after three months of intranasal vasopressin in healthy old humans.* Psychoneuroendocrinology, 1997. 22(6): p. 387-396.

[200] Koob, G.F., C. Lebrun, R.-M. Bluthé, R. Dantzer, and M. Le Moal, *Role of neuropeptides in earning versus performance: Focus on vasopressin.* Brain Research Bulletin, 1989. 23(4–5): p. 359-364.

[201] Le Moal, M., R. Dantzer, B. Michaud, and G.F. Koob, *Centrally injected arginine vasopressin (AVP) facilitates social memory in rats.* Neurosci. Lett., 1987. 77: p. 353-359.

[202] Jing, W., F. Guo, L. Cheng, J.-F. Zhang, and J.-S. Qi, *Arginine vasopressin prevents amyloid β protein-induced impairment of long-term potentiation in rat hippocampus in vivo.* Neuroscience Letters, 2009. 450(3): p. 306-310.

[203] Walum, H., L. Westberg, S. Henningsson, J.M. Neiderhiser, D. Reiss, W. Igl, J.M. Ganiban, E.L. Spotts, N.L. Pedersen, E. Eriksson, and P. Lichtenstein, *Genetic*

variation in the vasopressin receptor 1a gene (AVPR1A) associates with pair-bonding behavior in humans. Proceedings of the National Academy of Sciences, 2008. 105(37): p. 14153-14156.

[204] Bisceglia, R., J.M. Jenkins, K.G. Wigg, T.G. O'Connor, G. Moran, and C.L. Barr, *Arginine vasopressin 1a receptor gene and maternal behavior: evidence of association and moderation.* Genes, Brain and Behavior, 2012. 11(3): p. 262-268.

[205] Fries, A.B.W., T.E. Ziegler, J.R. Kurian, S. Jacoris, and S.D. Pollak, *Early experience in humans is associated with changes in neuropeptides critical for regulating social behavior.* Proceedings of the National Academy of Sciences of the United States of America, 2005. 102(47): p. 17237-17240.

[206] Dempster, E.L., I. Burcescu, K. Wigg, E. Kiss, I. Baji, J. Gadoros, Z. Tamás, K. Kapornai, G. Daróczy, J.L. Kennedy, A. Vetró, M. Kovacs, C.L. Barr, and D. The International Consortium for Childhood-Onset Mood, *Further genetic evidence implicates the vasopressin system in childhood-onset mood disorders.* European Journal of Neuroscience, 2009. 30(8): p. 1615-1619.

[207] Dempster, E.L., I. Burcescu, K. Wigg, E. Kiss, I. Baji, J. Gadoros, Z. Tamas, J.L. Kennedy, A. Vetro, M. Kovacs, C.L. Barr, and for the International Consortium for Childhood-Onset Mood Disorders, *Evidence of an Association Between the Vasopressin V1b Receptor Gene (AVPR1B) and Childhood-Onset Mood Disorders.* Arch Gen Psychiatry, 2007. 64(10): p. 1189-1195.

[208] Halbreich, U. and S. Karkun, *Cross-cultural and social diversity of prevalence of postpartum depression and depressive symptoms.* Journal of Affective Disorders, 2006. 91(2-3): p. 97-111.

[209] Hammen, C., *Stress and depression.* 2005. p. 293-319.

[210] Kirsch, I., B.J. Deacon, T.B. Huedo-Medina, A. Scoboria, T.J. Moore, and B.T. Johnson, *Initial Severity and Antidepressant Benefits: A Meta-Analysis of Data Submitted to the Food and Drug Administration.* PLoS Med, 2008. 5(2): p. e45.

[211] McGregor, I.S., P.D. Callaghan, and G.E. Hunt, *From ultrasocial to antisocial: a role for oxytocin in the acute reinforcing effects and long-term adverse consequences of drug use?* British Journal of Pharmacology, 2008. 154(2): p. 358-368.

[212] McGregor, I.S. and M.T. Bowen, *Breaking the loop: Oxytocin as a potential treatment for drug addiction.* Hormones and Behavior, 2012. 61(3): p. 331-339.

[213] Xue, Y.-X., Y.-X. Luo, P. Wu, H.-S. Shi, L.-F. Xue, C. Chen, W.-L. Zhu, Z.-B. Ding, Y.-p. Bao, J. Shi, D.H. Epstein, Y. Shaham, and L. Lu, *A Memory Retrieval-Extinction Procedure to Prevent Drug Craving and Relapse.* Science, 2012. 336(6078): p. 241-245.

[214] Zhou, Y., J.T. Bendor, V. Yuferov, S.D. Schlussman, A. Ho, and M.J. Kreek, *Amygdalar vasopressin mRNA increases in acute cocaine withdrawal: Evidence for opioid receptor modulation.* Neuroscience, 2005. 134(4): p. 1391-1397.

[215] Zhou, Y., F. Leri, E. Cummins, M. Hoeschele, and M.J. Kreek, *Involvement of Arginine Vasopressin and V1b Receptor in Heroin Withdrawal and Heroin Seeking Precipitated by Stress and by Heroin.* Neuropsychopharmacology, 2007. 33(2): p. 226-236.

[216] Edwards, S., M. Guerrero, O.M. Ghoneim, E. Roberts, and G.F. Koob, *Evidence that vasopressin V1b receptors mediate the transition to excessive drinking in ethanol-dependent rats.* Addiction Biology, 2012. 17(1): p. 76-85.

[217] Zimmerman, M., T. Sheeran, I. Chelminski, and D. Young, *Screening for psychiatric disorders in outpatients with DMS-IV substance use disorders.* J Subst Abuse Treat, 2004. 26: p. 181 - 188.

[218] Wolff, J.J., H. Gu, G. Gerig, J.T. Elison, M. Styner, S. Gouttard, K.N. Botteron, S.R. Dager, G. Dawson, A.M. Estes, A.C. Evans, H.C. Hazlett, P. Kostopoulos, R.C. McKinstry, S.J. Paterson, R.T. Schultz, L. Zwaigenbaum, and J. Piven, *Differences in White Matter Fiber Tract Development Present from 6 to 24 months in infants with autism.* American Journal of Psychiatry, 2012(1): p. 1-12.

[219] Modi, M.E. and L.J. Young, *The oxytocin system in drug discovery for autism: Animal models and novel therapeutic strategies.* Hormones and Behavior, 2012. 61(3): p. 340-350.

[220] Nephew, B.C. and R.S. Bridges, *Effects of chronic social stress during lactation on maternal behavior and growth in rats.* Stress, 2011. 14(6): p. 677-684.

Chapter 4

Role for Pituitary Neuropeptides in Social Behavior Disturbances of Schizophrenia

Tomiki Sumiyoshi, Tadasu Matsuoka and Masayoshi Kurachi

Additional information is available at the end of the chapter

http://dx.doi.org/10.5772/52326

1. Introduction

Derangement of hormonal milieu has been associated with the pathophysiology of psychiatric illnesses, such as schizophrenia, mood disorders, and developmental disorders [1; 2; 3]. Among them, schizophrenia is a relatively common neuropsychiatric disorder, and has been associated with debilitating consequences if not treated properly [4; 5]. The illness is characterized by positive (e.g., delusions, hallucinations, bizarre thoughts) and negative (blunt affect, avolition, anhedonia, social withdrawal) symptoms, as well as deficits in various cognitive abilities, e.g. verbal memory, working memory, attention/vigilance, and information processing [4; 6; 7]. Minor impairments of social cognition are often observed during the premorbid stage of the disease [8].

The role for endocrinological dysregulation in the development of psychotic symptoms has been suggested by brain imaging studies. For example, a larger than normal volume of the pituitary gland has been reported in patients with first-episode schizophrenia [9] (Fig. 1). Further, these patients exhibit an increase in the pituitary volume overtime, unlike the case with normal volunteers, the degree of which is correlated with the change in positive symptoms [9]. These findings, representing mainly a morphological change of the anterior pituitary [9], are consistent with the concept of HPA axis hyperactivity in response to stress during psychotic experience [10].

Hormones secreted from the posterior portion of the pituitary gland, i.e. vasopressin and oxytocin, have also been a focus in schizophrenia research from the perspective of social behavior disturbances [2; 11; 12]. In this chapter, we provide an overview of preclinical and clinical evidence for contribution of the vasopressin and oxytocin systems in social behavior deficits of schizophrenia and related disorders, as well as their treatment. Related discussions on the role of these neuropeptides in the coping of stressors and psychiatric conditions are provided in other Chapters [3; 13].

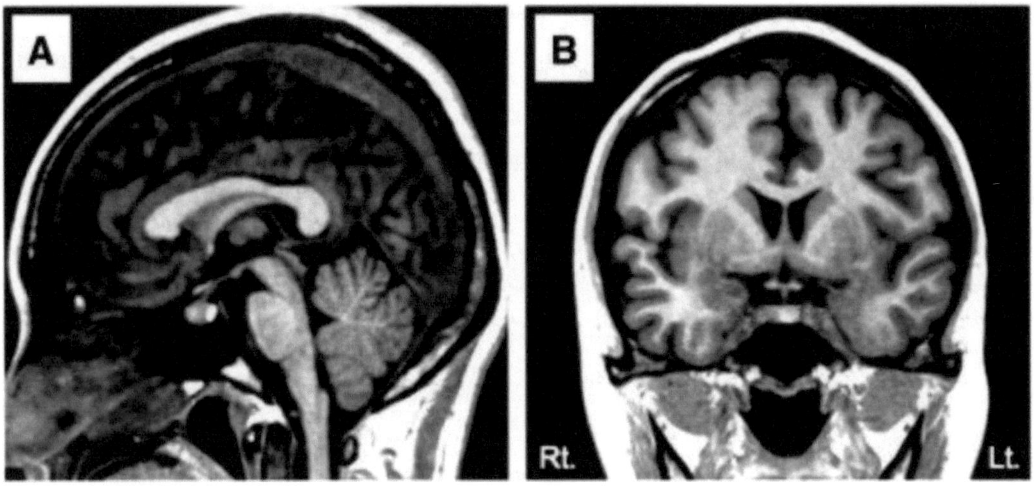

Figure 1. Sagittal (A) and coronal (B) views of the pituitary gland manually traced (in blue). The pituitary stalk was excluded from the tracings. (Takahashi T et al. *Prog Neuropsychopharmacol Biol Psychiatry* 35;177-83, 2011 (Permission obtained from Elsevier)

2. Vasopressin (arginine-vasopressin, AVP), oxytocin and behaviors

The two neuro-hormones are nona-peptides closely related each other, while their functions are sometimes in opposite directions, e.g. facial cognition and responses to stress [14]. Also, there is a suggestion that oxytocin is responsible for maternal behavior whereas male-typical social behavior is associated with AVP [2]. As a neuromodulator, AVP has been suggested to play a role in some of the cognitive abilities, including social memory, as well as emotionality (Fig 2). Neurotransmissions by AVP are mediated by three receptor subtypes, namely, V_{1A}, V_{1B}, and V_2 receptors, all of which are coupled to G-proteins [2]. Information about oxytocin is reviewed elsewhere in this Book [3]

Impaired social abilities have been particularly implicated in subjects with developmental disorders, such as autism. Thus, Fries et al (2005) [15] reported decreased urine levels of AVP and oxytocin, in children reared in orphanage settings compared to those in infants who received normal care-giving from their parents. Previously institutionalized children have been suggested to frequently experience problems in establishing social bonds and regulating social behavior [15]. Accordingly, infants who experienced early neglect showed lower basal levels of AVP than family-reared children [15]. These observations support the growing evidence for the role of the neuropeptidergic systems in social behaviors in mammals (e.g. [16; 17; 18]: see [19] for review).

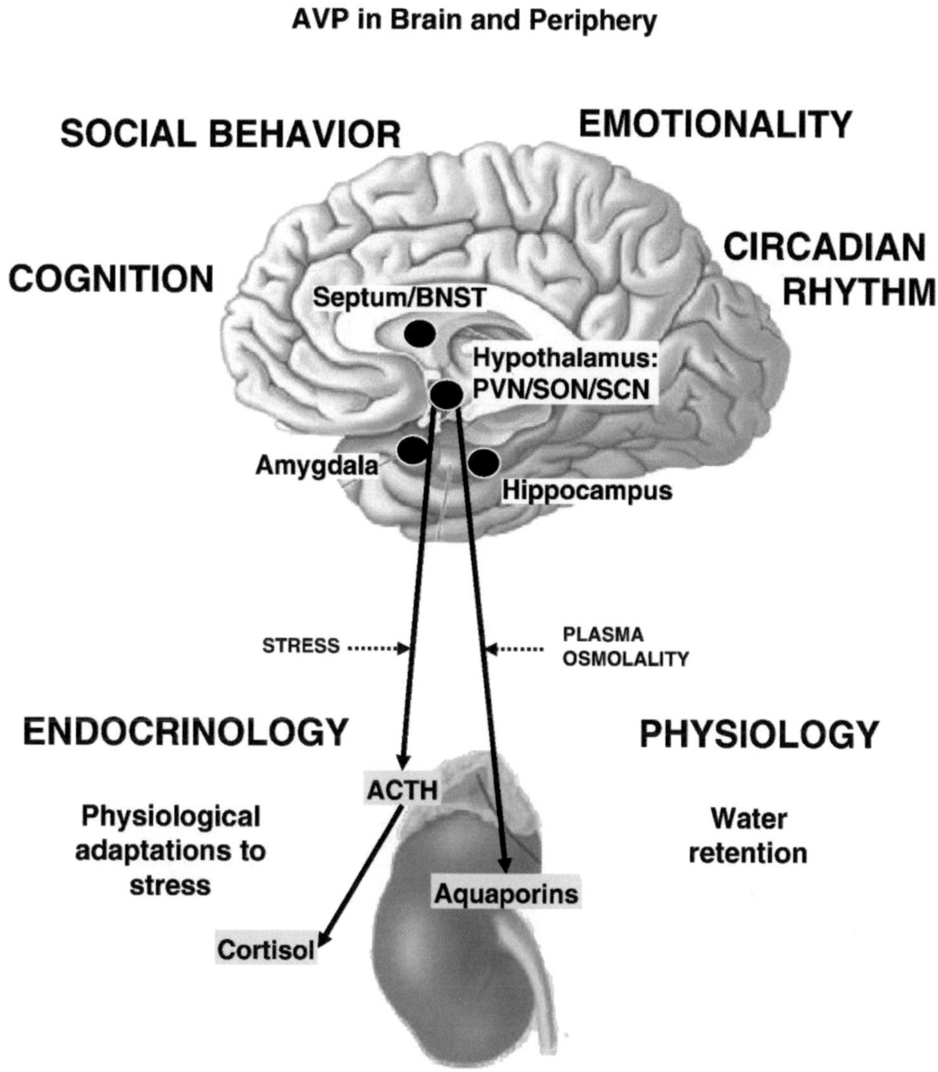

Figure 2. Arginine-vasopressin in the brain and periphery. Extracted from Frank E and Landgraf R. *Eur J Psychopharmacol* 583;226-42, 2008 (Permission obtained from Elsevier)

3. Sociality deficits in animal models of schizophrenia; Effect of neuropeptides

Social behaviors comprise various domains, such as social (learning) memory and social bonding [20; 21]. The intracerebroventricular administration of AVP has been shown to facilitate social memory, as measured by the social discrimination test (SDT), in rats [22; 23].

The neural substrates governing the ability of AVP to enhance sociality include the lateral septum (LS), bed nucleus of the stria terminalis, and medial amygdala [24]. Specifically, overexpression of the V_{1A} receptors in the LS enhanced SDT performance, an effect blocked

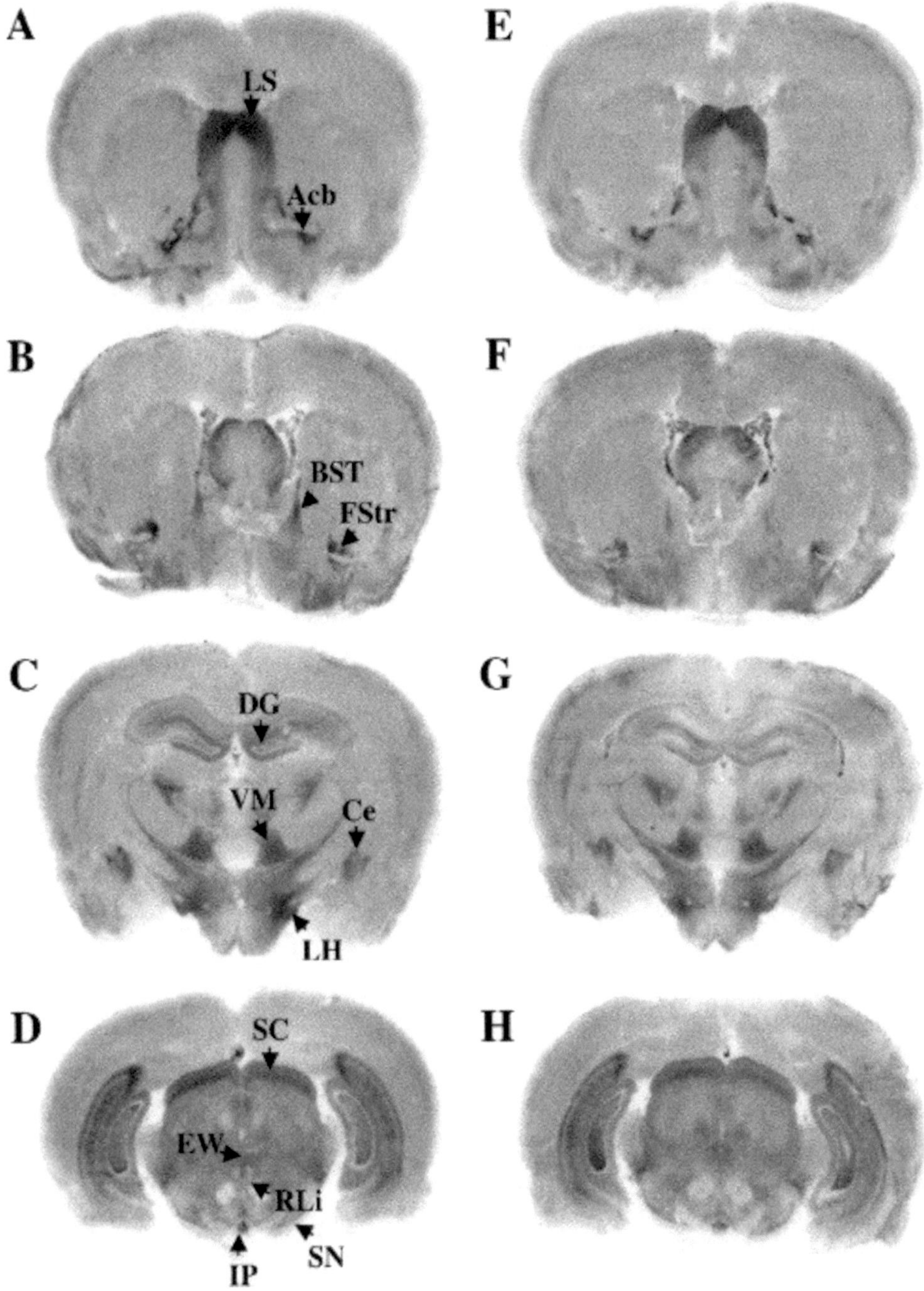

Figure 3. Autoradiographic localization of V1a receptor binding sites in coronal sections of the brain of the vehicle group (A–D) and PCP group (E–H) of rats with [^{125}I]-Linear AVP antagonist. Abbreviations: Acb, nucleus accumbens; FStr, fundus striati; LS, lateral septum; BST, bed nucleus of the stria terminalis; Ce, central amygdaloid nucleus; DG, dentate gyrus; VM, ventromedial thalamic nucleus; LH, lateral hypothalamic area; Rli, rostral linear raphe nucleus; SN, substantia nigra; IP, interpeduncular nucleus; SC, superior colliculus. Tanaka et al ., *Brain Res* 992; 239–245, 2003 (Permission obtained from Elsevier)

by application of a V_{1A} antagonist, but not oxytocin receptor antagonist [2]. By contrast, administration of oxytocin into the medial amygdala restored impaired social recognition in oxytocin knockout mice, while vasopressin was ineffective [25]. Overall, these observations are consistent with the contribution of V_1 receptors in the LS to the maintenance of long-term potentiation [26], which is crucial for learning and memory.

Experimental data from our laboratory also suggest a role for altered AVP transmissions in social interaction deficits. Thus, chronic administration of phencyclidine, an antagonist at N-methyl-D-aspartate (NMDA) receptors, impaired social interaction behavior, and reduced the density of V_{1A} receptors in several brain regions, including the LS in rats [18] (Figure 3). In a subsequent study, Matsuoka et al. (2008) [27] found decreased levels of mRNA encoding AVP in the amygdala, as measured by a microarray system and real-time quantitative PCR assay, in rats chronically treated with MK-801, a non-competitive antagonist at the NMDA receptor. These findings provide a basis for the ability of AVP or its analogues to ameliorate social interaction deficits in animal models of schizophrenia.

Accordingly, we reported that NC-1900, an AVP analogue and agonist at V1a receptors, ameliorates social interaction deficits in rats chronically treated with MK-801 [17] (Figure 4).

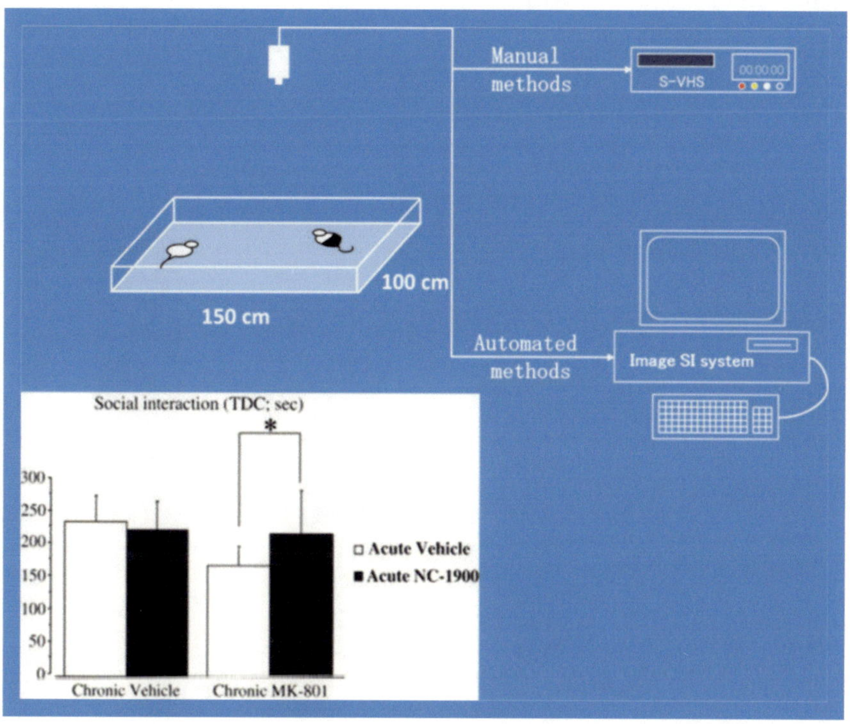

Figure 4. Measurement of social interaction behavior. A pair of rats (one dye-marked) are placed in an open arena, whose behavior, including "contact" (between-subject distance < 20 cm) is video-taped for manual viewing and/or automatically analyzed by a computer. (Inset)Total duration of contact (TDC) of rats during a 10-min observation period. Each bar represents mean ± SD of the time spent in social interaction (in seconds). *$P < 0.05$, chronic (MK-801, vehicle) × acute (NC-1900, vehicle) treatment interaction. Matsuoka et al. Brain Res 1053 (2005) 131-136. (Permission obtained from Elsevier).

This result from an animal model of schizophrenia is consistent with the observation, discussed above [18], that chronic administration of the NMDA antagonist phencyclidine reduces the density of V1a receptor binding sites in several brain regions, including the LS, in rats showing social interaction deficits. These findings from our laboratory are consistent with Bielsky et al [16] who reported that re-expressing of V1a receptors in the lateral septum of V1a receptor knockout mice exhibits complete recovery from impaired social recognition. Down-regulation of the AVP gene in the amygdala of MK-801-treated rats may provide a basis for the ability of AVP-analogues to ameliorate the behavioral disturbances by blockade of NMDA receptor [17]. Similar benefits regarding social behavior have been reported for oxytocin [3; 13; 28; 29; 30].

We conducted a further analysis of the change in the expression of RNAs encoding AVP and its receptor subtypes (V_{1A}, V_{1B}) in the amygdala of the model rat by means of qPCR (Table 1). As shown in Fig 5, expression of the AVP gene was significantly reduced by treatment with MK-801 (0.13 mg/day) for 14 days, while the same treatment did not affect the expressions of V_{1A}, and V_{1B} receptors. These results may help understand a mechanism by which impaired NMDA receptor-mediated transmissions, a putative pathophysiology of schizophrenia, disturbs social behaviors.

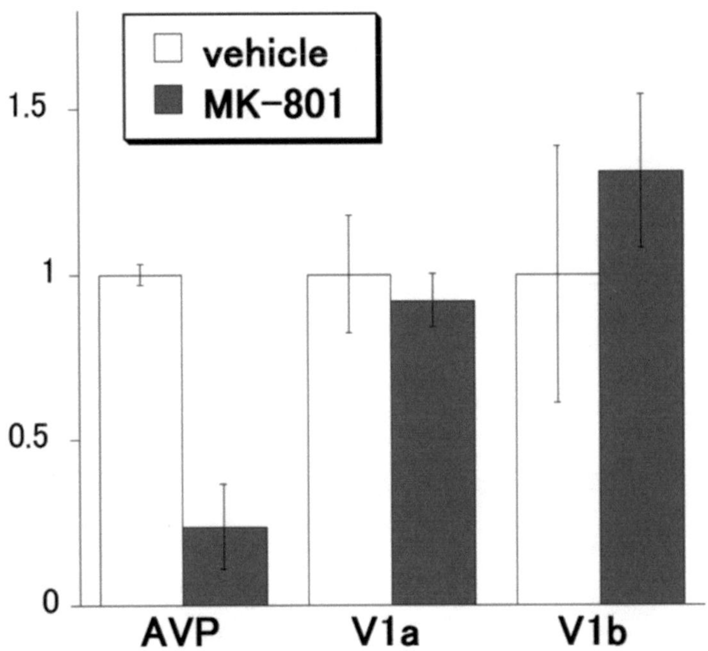

Figure 5. RNA quantification by means of real-time qPCR. Expression ratios for MK-801-treated rats vs. vehicle-treated animals are shown (n=5-6 for each group). Expression of the arginine-vasopressin (AVP) gene was significantly reduced by treatment with MK-801 (0.13 mg/day) for 14 days, (*$p<0.05$ by one-way ANOVA), while the same treatment did not affect the expressions of V1a and V1b receptors.Mx3000P (StrataGene) was used for pPCR with SYBER Premix Ex Taq (Takara Co. Ltd.). GAPDH was used as internal standard.

genes	forward	reverse	product size
GAPDH	tgaggaccaggttgtctcct	atgtaggccatgggtccac	162
AVP	acactacgctctctgcttg	cctcttgcctcctcttg	86
V1a	caaggatgactccgatagc	gatggatttggaagatttgg	112
V1b	ttctcagttgtgtggttcac	cctgtgcctttcagacttac	116

GAPDH, glyceraldehude-3-phosphate dehydrogenase.
AVP, arginine vasopressin. V1a, arginine vasopressin receptor 1a. V1b, vasopressin receptor 1b.

Table 1. Nucleotide sequences of RT-qPCR primers for target genes

4. Clinical implications

Efforts to enhance social ability are important from the perspective of adjusting patients to the community, thus improving functional outcome. Social ability disturbances in schizophrenia are thought to be partly attributable to negative symptoms and disturbances of cognitive function [4; 31; 32]. Although treatment with the first generation antipsychotic drugs, e.g. haloperidol, has been shown to ameliorate positive symptoms, only a limited number of agents, such as the second generation antipsychotics, or so-called "atypical antipsychotic drugs (AAPDs)", e.g. clozapine, melperone, risperidone, olanzapine, quetiapine, ziprasidone, and perospirone, with variable affinities for serotonin (5-HT) receptor subtypes, have been shown to be partially effective to treat negative symptoms and cognitive disturbances of schizophrenia [32; 33; 34; 35; 36] (see [4; 37] for review). Thus, more effective strategy to treat neurocognition, in addition to social abilities, is needed to enhance quality of life for patients.

In this context, the results from a recent study of the effect of augmentation therapy with oxytocin on cognitive function in patients with schizophrenia are noteworthy [38]. The investigators report a significant enhancement of verbal learning memory, a cognitive domain thought to largely influence the outcome, in subjects receiving daily intranasal oxytocin (twice daily) for 3 weeks. Further controlled study is warranted to confirm the cognition-boosting effect of neuropeptides in the treatment of schizophrenia.

As has been discussed, neuropeptides, e.g., vasopressin and oxytocin, have been suggested to be associated with the pathophysiology of schizophrenia. Accordingly, a whole-genome scan for schizophrenia in a large inbred Arab-Israeli pedigree has found a possible linkage on chromosome 20p13 [39] (Fig. 6). Importantly, this locus harbors four strong candidate genes for the illness, two of which are for oxytocin (*OXT*) and AVP (*AVP*) [39]. Further, examination of the association with gene expression in the brain identified genetic variants in the *OXT-AVP* cluster, and three of these variants were associated with schizophrenia [12]. These findings provide a strong proof for the contribution of these neuropeptides to the etiology of the illness.

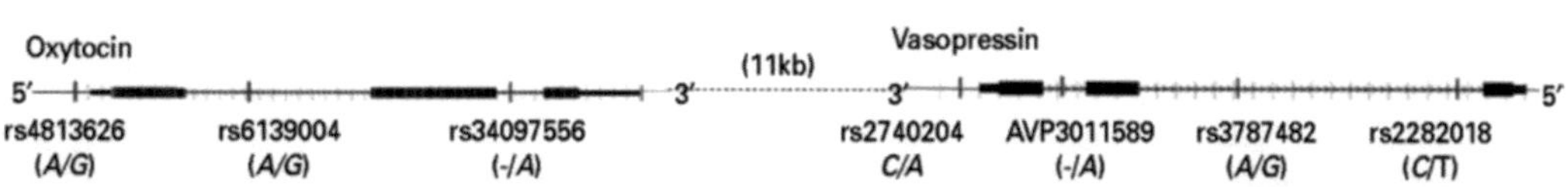

Figure 6. A scheme of the genes oxytocin and vasopressin on the chromosomal region 20p13 and the positions of the seven examined SNPs. Teltsh et al., *Int J Neuropsychopharmacol* 15;309-19, 2012 (Permission obtained from CINP).

5. Conclusions

Psychotropic drugs acting on 5-HT receptors, such as AAPDs and $5\text{-}HT_{1A}$ agonists, have been shown to improve social behavior in animals [36; 40; 41]. These results are consistent with the concept that the AVP and 5-HT systems interact both neuroanatomically and neurochemically in the brain areas, e.g. anterior hypothalamus, as demonstrated in Fig. 7 [42]. Therefore, it is reasonable that further research into the neuropeptidergic system, in conjunction with other neurotransmitter/modulator systems, will facilitate the therapeutic strategy for social behavior deficits in patients with schizophrenia and related disorders.

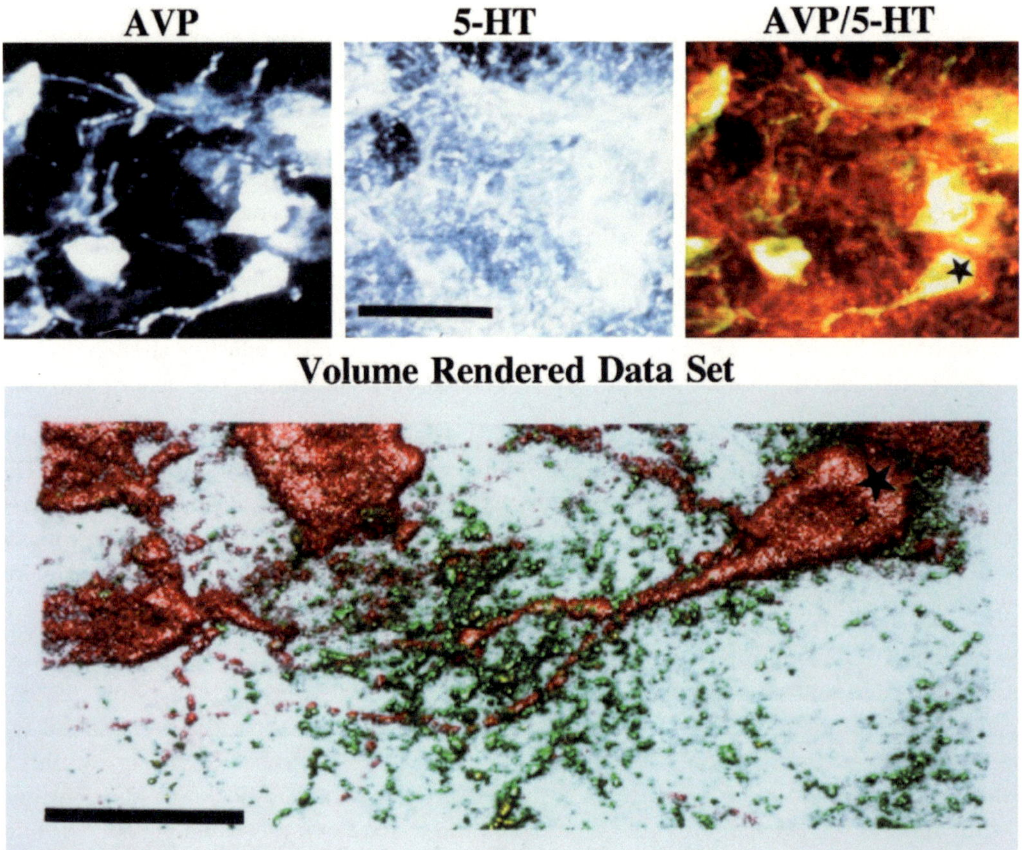

Figure 7. Photomicrographs of arginine vasopressin (AVP) and serotonin (5-HT), as revealed by double-labelling immunocytochemistry. Shown are AVP and 5-HT fluorescent immunoreactivity acquired through laser scanning confocal microscopy. The same single optical plane is shown for both neurochemical signals in the top black and white photographs. The combination of both digitized images is shown in color on the top right panel. The AVP is depicted in bright yellow and the 5-HT appears as a red/orange. A volume-rendered data set of serial optical sections through the AVP neuron denoted with the star is shown in the bottom color photograph. The green stippling is 5-HT varicosities and putative synapses clustered around the red-colored AVP neuron (denoted by the star). Scale bars: top, 50 μm; bottom, 30 μm. (Ferris C F et al. *J. Neurosci.* 1997;17:4331-43) (Permission obtained from the Society for Neuroscience)

Author details

Tomiki Sumiyoshi*, Tadasu Matsuoka and Masayoshi Kurachi
Department of Neuropsychiatry, University of Toyama Graduate School of Medicine and Pharmaceutical Sciences, Toyama, Japan

Acknowledgement

The authors declare no conflict of interest for this work.

We are grateful for fruitful discussions with Drs. Michio Suzuki, Tsutomu Takahashi and Kodai Tanaka.

This work was supported by Health and Labour Sciences Research Grants from Comprehensive Research on Disability, Health and Welfare, Grants-in—Aid for Scientific Research from the Japanese Society for the Promotion of Science, SENSHIN Medical Research Foundation, and Takeda Scientific Foundation.

6. References

[1] B.S. McEwen, E. Stellar, Stress and the individual. Mechanisms leading to disease. Arch Intern Med 153 (1993) 2093-2101.
[2] E. Frank, R. Landgraf, The vasopressin system--from antidiuresis to psychopathology. Eur J Pharmacol 583 (2008) 226-242.
[3] T. Munesue, K. Ashimura, H. Nakatani, M. Kikuchi, S. Yokoyama, M. Oi, H. Higashida, Y. Minabe, Is intranasal administration of oxytocin effective for social impairments in autism spectrum disorder? in: T. Sumiyoshi, (Ed.), Neuroendocrinology and Behavior, InTech, Rijeka, 2012, pp. ( ).
[4] T. Sumiyoshi, Y. Kawasaki, M. Suzuki, Y. Higuchi, M. Kurachi, Neurocognitive assessment and pharmacotherapy towards prevention of schizophrenia: What can we learn from first episode psychosis. Clin Psychopharmacol Neurosci 6 (2008) 57-64.
[5] C. Bouza, T. Lopez-Cuadrado, Z. Saz-Parkinson, R. Alcazar, J. Maria, A. Blanco, Natural mortality in schizophrenia: an updated meta-analysis, in: T. Sumiyoshi, (Ed.), Schizophrenia Research: Recent Advances, Nova Science Publishers, New York, 2012, pp. (61-80).
[6] Y. Kaneda, T. Sumiyoshi, R. Keefe, Y. Ishimoto, S. Numata, T. Ohmori, Brief assessment of cognition in schizophrenia: validation of the Japanese version. Psychiatry Clin Neurosci 61 (2007) 602-609.
[7] M. Matsui, T. Sumiyoshi, H. Arai, Y. Higuchi, M. Kurachi, Cognitive functioning related to quality of life in schizophrenia. Prog Neuropsychopharmacol Biol Psychiatry 32 (2008) 280-287.

* Corresponding Author

[8] L. Erlenmeyer-Kimling, D. Rock, S.A. Roberts, M. Janal, C. Kestenbaum, B. Cornblatt, U.H. Adamo, Gottesman, II, Attention, memory, and motor skills as childhood predictors of schizophrenia-related psychoses: the New York High-Risk Project. Am J Psychiatry 157 (2000) 1416-1422.

[9] T. Takahashi, S.Y. Zhou, K. Nakamura, R. Tanino, A. Furuichi, M. Kido, Y. Kawasaki, K. Noguchi, H. Seto, M. Kurachi, M. Suzuki, Longitudinal volume changes of the pituitary gland in patients with schizotypal disorder and first-episode schizophrenia. Prog in Neuro-Psychopharmacology & Biol Psychiat 35 (2011) 177-183.

[10] C.M. Pariante, K. Vassilopoulou, D. Velakoulis, L. Phillips, B. Soulsby, S.J. Wood, W. Brewer, D.J. Smith, P. Dazzan, A.R. Yung, I.M. Zervas, G.N. Christodoulou, R. Murray, P.D. McGorry, C. Pantelis, Pituitary volume in psychosis. J Psychiatry : 185 (2004) 5-10.

[11] T. Sumiyoshi, T. Matsuoka, K. Tanaka, V. Bubenikova-Valesova, Social interaction deficits in schizophrenia-spectrum disorders and pharmacologic intervention, in: A.T. Heatherton, V.A. Walcott, (Eds.), Handbook of Social Interactions in the 21st Century, Nova Science Publishers, New York, 2009, pp. 363-370.

[12] O. Teltsh, K. Kanyas-Sarner, A. Rigbi, L. Greenbaum, B. Lerer, Y. Kohn, Oxytocin and vasopressin genes are significantly associated with schizophrenia in a large Arab-Israeli pedigree. Int. Neuropsychopharmacol (2011) 1-11.

[13] B.C. Nephew, Behavioral roles of oxytocin and vasopressin, in: T. Sumiyoshi, (Ed.), Neuroendocrinology and Behavior, InTech, Rijeka, 2012, pp. (   ).

[14] M. Goldman, M. Marlow-O'Connor, I. Torres, C.S. Carter, Diminished plasma oxytocin in schizophrenic patients with neuroendocrine dysfunction and emotional deficits. Schizoph Res 98 (2008) 247-255.

[15] A.B. Fries, T.E. Ziegler, J.R. Kurian, S. Jacoris, S.D. Pollak, Early experience in humans is associated with changes in neuropeptides critical for regulating social behavior. Proc Natl Acad Sci U S A 102 (2005) 17237-17240.

[16] I.F. Bielsky, S.B. Hu, X. Ren, E.F. Terwilliger, L.J. Young, The V1a vasopressin receptor is necessary and sufficient for normal social recognition: a gene replacement study. Neuron 47 (2005) 503-513.

[17] T. Matsuoka, T. Sumiyoshi, K. Tanaka, M. Tsunoda, T. Uehara, H. Itoh, M. Kurachi, NC-1900, an arginine-vasopressin analogue, ameliorates social behavior deficits and hyperlocomotion in MK-801-treated rats: therapeutic implications for schizophrenia. Brain Res 1053 (2005) 131-136.

[18] K. Tanaka, M. Suzuki, T. Sumiyoshi, M. Murata, M. Tsunoda, M. Kurachi, Subchronic phencyclidine administration alters central vasopressin receptor binding and social interaction in the rat. Brain Res 992 (2003) 239-245.

[19] E.E. Storm, L.H. Tecott, Social circuits: peptidergic regulation of mammalian social behavior. Neuron 47 (2005) 483-486.

[20] D. de Wied, J.M. van Ree, Neuropeptides: animal behaviour and human psychopathology. Eur Arch Psychiatr Neurol Sci 238 (1989) 323-331.

[21] J.T. Winslow, N. Hastings, C.S. Carter, C.R. Harbaugh, T.R. Insel, A role for central vasopressin in pair bonding in monogamous prairie voles. Nature 365 (1993) 545-548.

[22] R. Dantzer, R.M. Bluthe, G.F. Koob, M. Le Moal, Modulation of social memory in male rats by neurohypophyseal peptides. Psychopharmacology 91 (1987) 363-368.

[23] M. Le Moal, R. Dantzer, B. Michaud, G.F. Koob, Centrally injected arginine vasopressin (AVP) facilitates social memory in rats. Neurosc Lett 77 (1987) 353-359.

[24] G.J. De Vries, R.M. Buijs, The origin of the vasopressinergic and oxytocinergic innervation of the rat brain with special reference to the lateral septum. Brain Res 273 (1983) 307-317.

[25] J.N. Ferguson, J.M. Aldag, T.R. Insel, L.J. Young, Oxytocin in the medial amygdala is essential for social recognition in the mouse. Neurosc 21 (2001) 8278-8285.

[26] M. Joels, Modulatory actions of steroid hormones and neuropeptides on electrical activity in brain. Eur J Pharmacol 405 (2000) 207-216.

[27] T. Matsuoka, M. Tsunoda, T. Sumiyoshi, I. Takasaki, Y. Tabuchi, T. Seo, K. Tanaka, T. Uehara, H. Itoh, M. Suzuki, M. Kurachi, Effect of MK-801 on gene expressions in the amygdala of rats. Synapse 62 (2008) 1-7.

[28] P.R. Lee, D.L. Brady, R.A. Shapiro, D.M. Dorsa, J.I. Koenig, Social interaction deficits caused by chronic phencyclidine administration are reversed by oxytocin. Neuropsychopharmacology 30 (2005) 1883-1894.

[29] P.R. Lee, D.L. Brady, R.A. Shapiro, D.M. Dorsa, J.I. Koenig, Prenatal stress generates deficits in rat social behavior: Reversal by oxytocin. Brain Res 1156 (2007) 152-167.

[30] D. Jin, H.X. Liu, H. Hirai, T. Torashima, T. Nagai, O. Lopatina, N.A. Shnayder, K. Yamada, M. Noda, T. Seike, K. Fujita, S. Takasawa, S. Yokoyama, K. Koizumi, Y. Shiraishi, S. Tanaka, M. Hashii, T. Yoshihara, K. Higashida, M.S. Islam, N. Yamada, K. Hayashi, N. Noguchi, I. Kato, H. Okamoto, A. Matsushima, A. Salmina, T. Munesue, N. Shimizu, S. Mochida, M. Asano, H. Higashida, CD38 is critical for social behaviour by regulating oxytocin secretion. Nature 446 (2007) 41-45.

[31] C. Sumiyoshi, T. Sumiyoshi, A. Roy, K. Jayathilake, H.Y. Meltzer, Atypical antipsychotic drugs and organization of long-term semantic memory: multidimensional scaling and cluster analyses of category fluency performance in schizophrenia. Int J Neuropsychopharmacol 9 (2006) 677-683.

[32] C. Sumiyoshi, A. Ertugrul, A.E. Anil Yagcioglu, Semantic memory deficits based on category fluency performance in schizophrenia: Similar impairment patterns of semantic organization across Turkish and Japanese patients. Psychiatry Res (2009)167:47-57..

[33] S.R. McGurk, The effect of clozapine on cognitive functioning in schizophrenia. J Clin Psychiatry 60 (suppl 12) (1999) 24-29.

[34] N.D. Woodward, S.E. Purdon, H.Y. Meltzer, D.H. Zald, A meta-analysis of neuropsychological change to clozapine, olanzapine, quetiapine, and risperidone in schizophrenia. Int J Neuropsychopharmacol 8 (2005) 457-472.

[35] T. Sumiyoshi, K. Jayathilake, H.Y. Meltzer, The effect of melperone, an atypical antipsychotic drug, on cognitive function in schizophrenia. Schizophr Res 59 (2003) 7-16.

[36] M. Bubenikova-Valesova, M. Votava, J. Palenicek, J. Horacek, C. Hoschl, Effect of serotonin-1A receptors on behavioral changes in animal model of schizophrenia-like behavior, in, 16th European Congress of Psychiatry, Nice, France, 2008.

[37] J. Horacek, V. Bubenikova-Valesova, M. Kopecek, T. Palenicek, C. Dockery, P. Mohr, C. Hoschl, Mechanism of action of atypical antipsychotic drugs and the neurobiology of schizophrenia. CNS Drugs 20 (2006) 389-409.

[38] D. Feifel, K. Macdonald, P. Cobb, A. Minassian, Adjunctive intranasal oxytocin improves verbal memory in people with schizophrenia. Schizoph Res 139 (2012) 207-210.

[39] O. Teltsh, K. Kanyas-Sarner, A. Rigbi, L. Greenbaum, B. Lerer, Y. Kohn, Oxytocin and vasopressin genes are significantly associated with schizophrenia in a large, Arab Israeli pedigree Int J Neuropsychopharmacol 15 (2012) 309-319.

[40] S. Snigdha, J.C. Neill, Improvement of phencyclidine-induced social behaviour deficits in rats: involvement of 5-HT1A receptors. Behav Brain Res 191 (2008) 26-31.

[41] R. Depoortere, A.L. Auclair, L. Bardin, L. Bruins Slot, M.S. Kleven, F. Colpaert, B. Vacher, A. Newman-Tancredi, F15063, a compound with D2/D3 antagonist, 5-HT_{1A} agonist and D_4 partial agonist properties. III. Activity in models of cognition and negative symptoms. Br J Pharmacol 151 (2007) 266-277.

[42] C.F. Ferris, R.H. Melloni, Jr., G. Koppel, K.W. Perry, R.W. Fuller, Y. Delville, Vasopressin/serotonin interactions in the anterior hypothalamus control aggressive behavior in golden hamsters. J Neurosci 17 (1997) 4331-4340.

Chapter 5

Is Intranasal Administration of Oxytocin Effective for Social Impairments in Autism Spectrum Disorder?

Toshio Munesue, Kazumi Ashimura, Hideo Nakatani, Mitsuru Kikuchi, Shigeru Yokoyama, Manabu Oi, Haruhiro Higashida and Yoshio Minabe

Additional information is available at the end of the chapter

http://dx.doi.org/10.5772/48798

1. Introduction

The neuropeptide oxytocin (OT) is synthesized in magnocellular neurons of the paraventricular and supraoptic nuclei of the hypothalamus and released from axon terminals in the neurohypophysis into the general circulation. However, OT is also released from somata and dendrites of magnocellular neurons into the brain [1]. OT release from axon terminals, somata and dendrites is regulated by not only activity-dependent Ca^{2+} influx, but also by mobilization of Ca^{2+} from intracellular Ca^{2+} stores [2, 3]. CD38, a transmembrane glycoprotein with ADP-ribosyl cyclase activity, plays a critical role in mobilization of intracellular Ca^{2+}, and therefore CD38 gene knockout ($CD38^{-/-}$) mice show low plasma OT concentrations [2]. On the other hand, CD38 is not responsible for the secretion of arginine vasopressin, which is another neurohypophyseal hormone [2].

Perioherally, OT promotes milk ejection in females and penile erection in males [4]. In addition, studies using OT gene knockout ($OT^{-/-}$), OT receptor gene knockout ($OTR^{-/-}$), or $CD38^{-/-}$ mice, in which OT signaling would be disrupted, were performed to investigate the roles of OT in the central nervous system [5, 6].

While $OT^{+/+}$ male mice showed a decline in the time investigating a female mouse during repeated pairings with full recovery following the introduction of a new female, $OT^{-/-}$ male mice show no such decline [7]. The results suggested that $OT^{-/-}$ male mice fail to develop social memory. Moreover, in a different experimental paradigm, $OT^{-/-}$ mice showed the same sociability, which was reflected as more time spent with a novel mouse as compared to time spent with a novel object, and preference for social novelty, which is reflected as more time spent with a second novel mouse as compared to time spent with a non-stranger mouse, as

$OT^{+/+}$ mice [8]. This experimental paradigm contains no memory component. Taken together, $OT^{-/-}$ mice exhibit impairments specific to social memory rather than deficits in general sociability. In addition, $OT^{-/-}$ infant mice show fewer call rates in ultrasonic vocalizations in response to maternal separation compared to $OT^{+/+}$ infant mice [9], so $OT^{-/-}$ mice may be less emotional in the mother-infant relationship.

When $OTR^{-/-}$ dams retrieve their infant mice scattered in the home gage, they take a longer time and spend less time crouching over infant mice than $OTR^{+/+}$ dams. $OTR^{-/-}$ infant mice show decreased ultrasonic vocalizations as seen in $OT^{-/-}$ infant mice [10]. While $OTR^{+/+}$ mice spend a longer time exploring a cage occupied by an unfamiliar mouse than an empty cage, $OTR^{-/-}$ mice spend the same time in exploring both cages [11]. Interestingly, forebrain-restricted $OTR^{-/-}$ male mice show a decline in the investigation time with the same female mice during repeated pairings and show full recovery following the introduction of a new female as with $OTR^{+/+}$ male mice [12].

$CD38^{-/-}$ male mice also show no decline in the investigation time with the same female mouse during repeated pairings unlike $CD38^{+/+}$ male mice [2]. $CD38^{-/-}$ infant mice show fewer call rates in ultrasonic vocalizations in response to maternal separation compared with $CD38^{+/+}$ infant mice [13].

$OT^{-/-}$, $OTR^{-/-}$, and $CD38^{-/-}$ mice show similar impairments in social memory and emotional relationship to the dam on isolation. Thus, investigations performed in OT-related knockout mice suggested the possible roles of OT as a sociability hormone. OT signaling in the brain was expected to play an important role in sociality in humans and to contribute to the etiologies of psychiatric disorders with social deficits, such as autism, which has been suggested to involve low plasma concentrations of OT [14].

Autism spectrum disorder (ASD) is a diagnostic continuum, which encompasses autistic disorder (autism), childhood disintegrative disorder, Asperger's disorder, and pervasive developmental disorder not otherwise specified in the Diagnostic and Statistical Manual of Mental Disorders (DSM) [15] and is intended to be designated so in a new version (DSM-5). Qualitative impairments of social interaction (social impairments) would be regarded as the major core symptom of ASD with repetitive and restrictive behaviors as another core symptom. However, social impairments imply wide-ranging symptoms from lack of declarative pointing, immediate echolalia, and failure to develop reciprocal peer relationships to very slight deficits identified only by detailed examinations combined with diagnostic tools, such as an advanced task for theory of mind [16]. Individuals with ASD, therefore, may not be diagnosed until adulthood [17].

While symptoms designated and conceptualized as impairments of social interaction are indispensable to the diagnosis of ASD and are easily identified in mentally retarded subjects with typical ASD, such as autism, weaker phenotypes of social impairments would involve a complicated subject of considering the symptomatology of ASD. Behavioral signs of social impairments in ASD have been suggested to emerge as a decline in social engagement, such as gazing on faces and social smiles, between 6 and 12 months of age [18]. These results imply that ASD is a nearly innate rather than acquired disease, although it could not be excluded that exogenous factors may exert adverse effects on newborns within the 6 months after birth. However, the clear boundary between the conditions with and without ASD could not be defined in research or from a clinical perspective. Autistic traits in the general population are common and show a continuous distribution [19]. Moreover, the symptom of social impairment has a different meaning in nature compared to all other medical symptoms. A fasting blood sugar level of 150 mg/dL in an individual with diabetes mellitus is an objective and independent measurement. Social impairments in an individual with ASD are by no means objective and independent, especially in the boundary region between the conditions with and without ASD. The term "social" has relevance to human "society." Human society is the whole that has been shaped by innumerably iterated social interactions among humans from time immemorial, and cannot be defined from an external standpoint. While behaviors exhibited by individuals with ASD may look more or less deviant from the viewpoint of human society, they adapt themselves to human society unremarkably in some cases and deviate from it directly in other cases. Social impairments in ASD subjects cannot be anchored exactly in the context of real-life environments. Therefore, it is very difficult to determine how symptoms of social impairment should be evaluated in treatment of patients with ASD.

In this article, we first discuss the influence of intranasally administered OT on sociality in human adults. We further examine the results obtained from four studies in which the effectiveness of intranasally or intravenously administered OT was investigated in ASD subjects. Moreover, we discuss long-term clinical trials in progress, for which we searched the public databases, of intranasally administered OT in subjects with ASD in randomized, double-blind, placebo-controlled designs. Finally, we consider the improvements in social impairments in the treatment of patients with ASD.

2. Effectiveness of intranasally administered OT on social cognition and prosocial behaviors in healthy adults

We consider that reciprocal interaction with others would go through the processes of self-consciousness as a construct deeply embedded in human society, social cognition, and prosocial behavior. Self-consciousness (i.e., self-representation or self-reference) may be a key concept in considering the psychopathology of ASD [20]. Can individuals with attenuated self-consciousness distinguish self from others in a social context? Children and adolescents with ASD made fewer statements classified as the social not but physical, active and psychological category compared to non-ASD subjects [21]. Typical interaction with others may be realized only under the conditions of typical self-consciousness. While biological investigations of self-consciousness have been performed using functional magnetic resonance imaging in ASD and healthy individuals [22, 23], the effects of OT on self-consciousness in humans remain unclear.

Social cognition implies important factors underlying not just face-to-face exchanges with others but also even circumstances alone in a crowd. People may wonder "Who is he?" "What has my daughter been thinking?" or "That person is watching me". All of this corresponds to social cognition. Prosocial behavior implies the favorable or unfavorable impressions that a person has toward others, and the following actions based on these impressions. People are impressed by others' behaviors and may bring these impressions into actions: "He looks trustworthy. I will consult with him about which course to take after graduation," "I hate people who discriminate against the weak. So, I will not talk to him." These are prosocial behaviors.

There have been many studies regarding the effects of OT on social cognition and prosocial behavior in healthy adults since the pioneering study by Kosfeld et al. [24] Interest in OT has increased due to the positive results obtained: e.g., strengthening of memory for faces [25] and increased emotional empathy [26] in social cognition, increased generosity [27] and trust [28] in prosociality. However, the results are inconsistent on closer inspection (for details, see [29]). For example, 259 healthy students participated in a study regarding the effects of OT on cooperative behavior in a randomized, double-blind, placebo-controlled design [30]. Participants played two economic games, which were a Coordination Game with strong incentives to cooperate and a Prisoner's Dilemma game with weak cooperative incentives, after one-half of them talked together and the other half spoke to no-one. The former group receiving OT showed more cooperation only in the Coordination Game than participants receiving placebo. However, the latter group receiving OT showed less cooperation only in the Cooperation Game than participants receiving placebo. Prosocial behaviors on receiving OT proceeded in the opposite directions according to whether social information was presented previously.

Based on the review of Bartz et al. [29], of 14 studies investigating social cognition, nine (69.2%) showed that OT exerted a significant main effect on the outcome compared to placebo (Table 1). Eight of these nine studies suggested that the effect of OT was significantly modulated by situational differences or individual factors. However, there was a marginal trend between the distributions of two categorical variables of OT effect and modulated OT effect (Fisher's exact test, $P = 0.095$).

			Modulated oxytocin effect		Fisher's exact test
			Yes	No	
Social cognition	Oxytocin effect	Significant	8	1	P = 0.095
		Null	2	3	
Prosociality	Oxytocin effect	Significant	5	12	P = 0.006
		Null	12	3	

Table 1. Relationship between oxytocin effect and modulated oxytocin effect (designed according to [25])

Of 32 studies investigating prosocial behavior, 17 (53.1%) showed that OT exerted a significant main effect on the outcome compared to placebo. Five of these 17 studies suggested that the effect of OT was significantly modulated by situational differences or individual factors. On the other hand, 12 of 15 studies without a significant main effect of OT were significantly modulated by situational differences or individual factors. The distribution of two categorical variables was significantly different ($P = 0.006$). The more these factors affect study participants, the less the effects of OT emerge in them. That is, the effects of OT on sociality, especially prosocial behavior, may be affected by external factors in addition to the function of OT itself and, moreover, external factors may show paradoxical effects. For example, 66 healthy adults participated in a money game, in which they rated their emotions (envy and gloating) toward their opponents when they gained more or less money, in double-blind, placebo-controlled, with-in subject design [31]. Interestingly, OT increased the envy ratings when the participant gained less money and the gloating ratings when they gained more money compared to placebo.

While early research that suggested effectiveness of OT in psychiatric diseases such as social anxiety disorder and ASD generated considerable enthusiasm, the reasons for the inconsistent and paradoxical results of OT on sociality in healthy humans remain unresolved. However, the pathophysiology of ASD has not yet been elucidated and no effective treatments for social impairments in ASD exist. It would be useful to investigate whether OT can improve the core symptoms of ASD.

3. Effectiveness of intranasally or intravenously administered OT in ASD subjects

Four randomized, double-blind, placebo-controlled trials of short-term OT administration in subjects with high-functioning ASD have been published since 2003 (Table 2) [32−35].

Reference number	n	Male gender	Age (years)	Intelligence quotient	Medication method	Oxytocin dose	Outcomes
32	15	14	19−56	74−110	Intravenously	10U	Repetitive behavior scale
33	15	14	19−56	74−110	Intravenously	10U	Comprehension of affective speech
34	13	11	17−39	unknown	Intranasally	24 IU	Social ball tossing game
35	16	16	12−19	unknown	Intranasally	18 or 24 IU	Reading the Mind in the Eyes-Revised

Table 2. Randomized, double-blind, placebo-controlled trials of short-term oxytocin administration in subjects with high-functioning autism spectrum disorder

The designs were naturally different between these studies in terms of age and gender of participants, medication methods, doses of OT and outcomes, so no conclusions could be drawn regarding the treatment of ASD patients based on a single-dose design. However, OT may play a role in alleviating repetitive symptoms [32] and modifying social impairments [33−35].

With regard to social impairments, Hollander et al. investigated the effectiveness of intravenously administered OT on comprehension of affective speech in 15 subjects with ASD in a randomized, double-blind, placebo-controlled, cross-over design [33]. The task was fairly easy for the participants resulting in the same improvements of scores of those who were administered placebo in the first condition as those who were administered OT in the first condition. However, after an interval between the first and second conditions (days: mean = 16.07; SD = 14.26), the scores at baseline in the second condition were retained in the participants administered OT and dropped in those administered placebo. These results suggested that OT may play a role in social memory acquisition in social cognition in ASD subjects.

Andari et al. investigated the effectiveness of intranasally administered OT on trust and preference toward opponent players using a social ball tossing game in 13 subjects with ASD by randomized, double-blind, placebo-controlled, within-subject design [34] (No results of face perception tasks shown in the study are noted here). ASD subjects administered OT trusted more and showed stronger preference for good than bad opponent players regardless of the perception of monetary rewards. No significant differences were found under placebo conditions. These results suggest that OT may play a role in prosocial behavior in subjects with ASD. Moreover, it was noted that plasma OT concentration at 10 min after nasal administration of OT show a significant increase compared to baseline concentration.

Guastella et al. investigated the effectiveness of intranasally administered OT on emotion recognition using the Reading the Mind in the Eyes Test-Revised [36] in 16 subjects with ASD by randomized, double-blind, placebo-controlled, cross-over design [35]. The improved performance by OT compared to placebo was restricted to the younger participants aged 12 to 15 and easy items in the test. These results suggest that OT may play a role in emotion recognition in social cognition for ASD subjects, although age and task difficulty may act as modulators.

Taken together, short-term (continuous intravenous infusion over 4 h or nasal spray of certain doses at a time) administration of OT may show effectiveness on social cognition and prosocial behavior in ASD subjects with situational differences or individual factors as confounders taken into account. The next step should be to investigate whether long-term administration of OT modulates social impairments in ASD.

4. Long-term randomized, double-blind, placebo-controlled trials of OT in subjects with ASD registered in the public databases

We searched the public databases, i.e., Clinicaltrials.gov (http://clinicaltrials.gov), UMIN Clinical Trials Registry (http://www.umin.ac.jp/ctr/index-j.htm), and Australian New Zealand Clinical Trials Registry (http://www.anzctr.org.au/), for long-term clinical trials of OT in ASD. In other databases of EU Clinical Trials Register (https://www.clinicaltrialsregister.eu/) and ISRCTN Register (http://www.isrctn.org/), we could not obtain the detailed information about long-term clinical trials of OT in ASD.

Nine pioneering clinical trials are in progress (Table 3). Although there is considerable diversity in age and gender of participants, oxytocin doses and trial duration, primary and secondary outcome measures would be the most noticeable items and are discussed here.

Registered identifier	Registered date	Estimated enrollment	Age (years)	Gender	Intellectual disability
NCT01417026	11 August 2011	68	12−17	Male	Profound mental retardation excluded
NCT01337687	10 December 2010	34	18−55	Both	Excluded
NCT01256060	22 November 2010	84	12−18	Both	Excluded
UMIN000003812	7 January 2010	20	10−14	Male	Not excluded
UMIN000005211	8 March 2011	60	>15	Both	Excluded
UMIN000007122	1 February 2012	20	18−54	Male	Excluded
UMIN000007250	9 February 2012	30	15−44	Male	Restricted to subjects with intellectual disability
ACTRN12611000061932	17 January 2011	40	3−8	Both	Not excluded
ACTRN12609000513213	29 June 2009	40	12−18	Male	Excluded

Registered number	Oxytocin doses per day	Oxytocin duration	Primary and secondary outcome measures
NCT01417026	24 IU	5 days	Part/Whole Identity Test, Reading the Mind in the Eyes Test,social attention, reward/motivation, perception, and cognition tasks
NCT01337687	48 IU	8 weeks	Clinical Global Impressions Scale- Severity and Improvement. Yale Brown Obsessive Compulsive Scale, Repetitive Behavior Scale−Revised, Diagnostic Analysis of Nonverbal Accuracy−2
NCT01256060	0.8 IU / kg	12 weeks	Diagnostic Analysis of Nonverbal Accuracy, Social Responsiveness Scale, Clinical Global Impressions Scale−Improvement, Repetitive Behavior Scale−Revised, Child Yale-Brown Obsessive-Compulsive Scale
UMIN000003812	Maximum 24 IU	12 months	Child Behavior Checklist, Autism Diagnostic Observation Schedule, Childhood Autism Rating Scale
UMIN000005211	Unknown	Unknown	Aberrant Behavior Checklist, Childhood Autism Rating Scale, Zung Self-Rating Depression Scale, State-Trait Anxiety Inventory
UMIN000007122	48 IU	6 weeks	Autism Diagnostic Observation Schedule, Childhood Autism Rating Scale 2, Psychological paradigms to test social cognition and behavior
UMIN000007250	16 IU	8 weeks	Childhood Autism Rating Scale, Clinical Global Impressions, Aberrant Behavior Checklist, Global Assessment of Functioning, Interaction Rating Scale Advanced
ACTRN12611000061932	Maximum 12 IU	5 weeks	Positive social interaction, Severity of repetitive behavior, Clinical Global Impressions, Preferential attention to social stimuli, Developmental Behavior Checklist, Social behavior scale
ACTRN12609000513213	12−18 IU	8 weeks	Social Responsiveness Scale, Reading the Mind in the Eyes Test, Repetitive Behavior Scale, Clinician Global Assessment

Table 3. Randomized, double-blind, placebo-controlled trials of intranasally short-term oxytocin administration in subjects with high-functioning autism spectrum disorder based on the public databases

The Social Responsiveness Scale provides quantitative measurements of social impairments in ASD by assessing domain of sociality such as social awareness and social information processing [37], and has been used as an outcome measure for interventions [38, 39]. The Reading the Mind in the Eyes Test [36] measures an aspect of social cognition by having the subjects assess emotion through the look of an actor's eye in photographs and has been adopted in many experimental trials [35, 40]. The Diagnostic Analysis of Nonverbal Accuracy Scale measures receptive and expressive abilities for receiving and sending emotions in faces, gestures, postures, and prosody [41], and has been used in the researches of not only ASD [42] but also of other mental disorders [43]. The Childhood Autism Rating Scale helps to identify subjects with ASD and determine symptom severity and has been commonly used in research and clinical settings. The scale assesses various domains of symptoms in ASD, including social impairments. The Autism Diagnostic Observation Schedule is a tool for assessment of symptoms of ASD through structured and semi-structured activities with subjects and provides scores in communication, social, and restricted and repetitive domains [44]. This tool has been regarded as the gold standard for assessing and diagnosing ASD. The Interaction Rating Scale Advanced assesses a practical index of social skills using five-minute video recorded interaction session [45]. It is interesting to note that this new tool may provide a validated measure of social impairments of ASD. The evaluations mentioned above provide quantitative values of social impairments of ASD based on caregivers' self-reports or behavioral observations.

At present, there is no commonly used assessment of symptoms in ASD, especially social and communication domains, for any interventions in contrast to the Positive and Negative Symptom Scale in schizophrenia and Hamilton Rating Scale for Depression in major depressive disorder, which are widely used as almost definitive measures. In the well-known research in which risperidone, a second-generation antipsychotic, was shown to be effective for reduction of irritability in subjects with ASD, the authors stated that they were unable to identify a validated measure for the core symptoms of ASD, i.e., social impairments [46].

A key question is whether these outcome measures could be used to sensitively assess improvements in sociality, which may only be subtle changes. This question remains unanswered before publication of the results of these trials.

5. What are the improvements of social impairments in the treatments of patients with ASD?

Social impairments in ASD have fundamentally different meanings from personality characteristics, such as introversion, interpersonal tension, or aloofness. Infants or preschool children with ASD may indicate very unique and impressive behaviors in the social context, which substantially reflect the disparity between typically developing children and children with ASD in social interaction. Here, we will describe pointing behaviors as an illustration.

When one points at something, others are invariably around. When one points at something, one invariably attempts to convey any information to others around. A toddler pulls his/her mother's sleeve, points to a miniature car on a shelf, and then looks at his/her mother's face (requesting pointing). When a preschool child sees a rainbow in the sky after rain, he/she runs up to his/her mother, takes her to the garden, and points to the rainbow while looking at her (declarative pointing). Liszkowski et al. found that twelve-month-old infants show different attitudes according to experimenter's reactions when infants point declaratively [47]. When experimenters responded to infants' declarative pointing but attended an incorrect referent with positive attitude, infants repeated pointing to redirect the experimenters' attention. When experimenters identified the correct referent with negative attitude, infants did not repeat pointing. When experimenters identified the correct referent and shared interest in it, infants appeared satisfied. Pointing is a prototypical behavior of interpersonal exchange, i.e., sociality.

Toddlers with ASD display a reduced incidence of declarative pointing compared to typically developing toddlers [48]. Declarative pointing constitutes a significantly diagnostic sign as well as social interest and joint attention for early detection of ASD [49]. Individuals with ASD have an innate disability in the social domain.

We consider that it would be essential to refer to one's own self and others if social impairments in ASD are discussed, because our own selves are embedded in a society full of others [20]. Individuals with ASD may be unable to mentalize the inner states of typically developing individuals, and this raises the question of whether typically developing individuals can mentalize the inner states of individuals with ASD. "Theory of mind" tasks would be regarded as tasks in ASD with "altered" self-consciousness proposed by individuals with "intact" self-consciousness.

According to the standpoint of traditional German psychopathology, self-consciousness (Ichbesstsein in German) is formally comprised of four prototypical representations. First, one's own self is identical at all times. Second, one's own self is always consistent. Third, all of one's own acts belong to one's own self. Finally, one's own self differs from others' own self. These representations deeply embedded in social interactions are intrinsically self-evident and underlie interpersonal exchange of sociality. While one exists almost without reflection on these representations in daily life, severe disruption of self-consciousness would have fairly serious consequences, such as dissociative identity crisis, doppelganger, xenopathic experiences and delusions of possession. Interestingly, children with ASD performed significantly less well on the self-test question than the other-person test question using tasks in which participants have to reflect an awareness of one's own prior belief [50]. These results suggest that individuals with ASD represent altered self-consciousness as mentioned above: "all of one's own acts belong to one's own self."

Although self-consciousness have been investigated using functional magnetic resonance imaging in ASD and healthy individuals [22, 23], the effects of OT on self-consciousness in humans have not been examined.

It is essential but difficult to answer questions regarding improvements of social impairments associated with treatment of patients with ASD. However, it may be useful to assess self-consciousness, although there is as yet no suitable test to examine representations of self-consciousness available in ASD research.

6. Conclusion

We hypothesized that OT signaling in the central nervous system may play a significant role in the pathophysiology of ASD based on studies using OT-related knockout mice, effectiveness in social context of OT to healthy subjects, and the results of short-term administration of OT on social impairments in ASD subjects. Long-term clinical trials of OT in ASD subjects are currently in progress. It is difficult to determine how symptoms of social impairment should be assessed in interventions in patients with ASD, although investigation of self-consciousness may provide important insights regarding this issue.

Author details

Toshio Munesue, Kazumi Ashimura, Mitsuru Kikuchi, Shigeru Yokoyama, Manabu Oi and Haruhiro Higashida
Research Center for Child Mental Development, Kanazawa University, Kanazawa, Japan

Hideo Nakatani
Department of Psychiatry and Neurobiology, Graduate School of Medical Science, Kanazawa university, Kanazawa, Japan

Yoshio Minabe
Research Center for Child Mental Development, Kanazawa University, Kanazawa, Japan
Department of Psychiatry and Neurobiology, Graduate School of Medical Science, Kanazawa University, Kanazawa, Japan

Acknowledgement

We are grateful for funding by the Strategic Research Program for Brain Sciences of the Ministry of Education, Culture, Sports, Science, and Technology of Japan for the long-term clinical trial of OT in patients with ASD (Registered identifier UMIN00007250 in Table 3).

7. References

[1] Ludwig M, Leng G (2006) Dendritic Peptide Release and Peptide-Dependent Behaviours. Nat. rev. neurosci. 7: 126-136.
[2] Jin D, Liu HX, Hirai H, Torashima T, Nagai T, Lopatina O, Shnayder NA, Yamada K, Noda M, Seike T, Fujita K, Takasawa S, Yokoyama S, Koizumi K, Shiraishi Y, Tanaka S, Hashii M, Yoshihara T, Higashida K, Islam MS, Yamada N, Hayashi K, Noguchi N, Kato I, Okamoto H, Matsushima A, Salmina A, Munesue T, Shimizu N, Mochida S, Asano M, Higashida H (2007) CD38 is Critical for Social Behaviour by Regulating Oxytocin Secretion. Nature. 446: 41-45.

[3] Tobin VA, Douglas AJ, Leng G, Ludwig M (2011) The Involvement of Voltage-Operated Calcium Channels in Somato-Dendritic Oxytocin Release. PLoS one. 6: e25366.

[4] Argiolas A, Melis MR (2005) Central Control of Penile Erection: Role of the Paraventricular Nucleus of the Hypothalamus. Prog. neurobiol. 76: 1-21.

[5] Higashida H, Yokoyama S, Kikuchi M, Munesue T (2012) CD38 and its Role in Oxytocin Secretion and Social Behavior. Horm. behav. 61: 351-358.

[6] Higashida H, Lopatina O, Yoshihara T, Pichugina YA, Soumarokov AA, Munesue T, Minabe Y, Kikuchi M, Ono Y, Korshunova N, Salmina AB (2010) Oxytocin Signal and Social Behaviour: Comparison among Adult and Infant Oxytocin, Oxytocin Receptor and CD38 Gene Knockout Mice. J. neuroendocrinol. 22: 373-379.

[7] Ferguson JN, Young LJ, Hearn EF, Matzuk MM, Insel TR, Winslow JT (2000) Social Amnesia in Mice Lacking the Oxytocin Gene. Nat. genet. 25: 284-288.

[8] Crawley JN, Chen T, Puri A, Washburn R, Sullivan TL, Hill JM, Young NB, Nadler JJ, Moy SS, Young LJ, Caldwell HK, Young WS (2007) Social Approach Behaviors in Oxytocin Knockout Mice: Comparison of Two Independent Lines Tested in Different Laboratory Environments. Neuropeptides, 41: 145-163.

[9] Winslow JT, Hearn EF, Ferguson J, Young LJ, Matzuk MM, Insel TR (2000) Infant Vocalization, Adult Aggression, and Fear Behavior of an Oxytocin Null Mutant Mouse. Horm. behav. 37: 145-155.

[10] Takayanagi Y, Yoshida M, Bielsky IF, Ross HE, Kawamata M, Onaka T, Yanagisawa T, Kimura T, Matzuk MM, Young LJ, Nishimori K (2005) Pervasive Social Deficits, but Normal Parturition, in Oxytocin Receptor-Deficient Mice. Proc. natl. acad. sci. u s a. 102: 16096-16101.

[11] Sala M, Braida D, Lentini D, Busnelli M, Bulgheroni E, Capurro V, Finardi A, Donzelli A, Pattini L, Rubino T, Parolaro D, Nishimori K, Parenti M, Chini B (2011) Pharmacologic Rescue of Impaired Cognitive Flexibility, Social Deficits, Increased Aggression, and Seizure Susceptibility in Oxytocin Receptor Null Mice: A Neurobehavioral Model of Autism. Biol. psychiatry. 69: 875-882.

[12] Lee HJ, Caldwell HK, Macbeth AH, Tolu SG, Young WS 3rd (2008) A Conditional Knockout Mouse Line of the Oxytocin Receptor. Endocrinology. 149: 3256-3263.

[13] Liu HX, Lopatina O, Higashida C, Tsuji T, Kato I, Takasawa S, Okamoto H, Yokoyama S, Higashida H (2008) Locomotor Activity, Ultrasonic Vocalization and Oxytocin Levels in Infant CD38 Knockout Mice. Neurosci. lett. 448: 67-70.

[14] Modahl C, Green L, Fein D, Morris M, Waterhouse L, Feinstein C, Levin H (1998) Plasma Oxytocin Levels in Autistic Children. Biol. psychiatry. 43: 270-277.

[15] American Psychiatric Association (2000) Diagnostic and Statistical Manual of Mental Disorders, Fourth Edition, Text Revision. Washington, D. C.: American Psychiatric Association.

[16] Baron-Cohen S, Jolliffe T, Mortimore C, Robertson M (1997) Another Advanced Test of Theory of Mind: Evidence from Very High Functioning Adults with Autism or Asperger Syndrome. J child. psyhcol. psychiatry. 38: 813-822.

[17] Bankier B, Lenz G, Gutierrez K, Bach M, Katschnig H (1999) A Case of Asperger's Syndrome First Diagnosed in Adulthood. Psychopathology. 32: 43-46.

[18] Ozonoff S, Iosif AM, Baguio F, Cook IC, Hill MM, Hutman T, Rogers SJ, Rozga A, Sangha S, Sigman M, Steinfeld MB, Young GS (2010) A Prospective Study of the Emergence of Early Behavioral Signs of Autism. J. am. acad. child adolesc. psychiatry. 49: 256-266.
[19] Constantino JN, Todd RD (2003) Autistic Traits in the General Population: A twin study. Arch. gen. psychiatry. 60: 524-530.
[20] Lombardo MV, Baron-Cohen S (2011) The Role of the Self in Mindblindness in Autism. Conscious. cong. 20: 130-140.
[21] Lee A, Hobson RP (1998) On Developing Self-concepts: A Controlled Study of Children and Adolescents with Autism. J. child psycho. psychiatry. 39: 1131-1144.
[22] Lombard MV, Chakrabarti B, Bullmore ET, Sadek SA, Pasco G, Wheelwright SJ, Suckling J, MRC AIMS Consortium, Baron-Cohen S (2010) Atypical Neural Self-Representation in Autism. Brain. 133: 611-624.
[23] Gusnard DA, Akbudak E, Shulman GL, Raichle ME (2001) Medial Prefrontal Cortex and Self-Referential Mental Activity: Realtion to a Default Mode of Brain function. Proc. natl. acad. sci. u s a. 98: 4259-4264.
[24] Kosfeld M, Heinrichs M, Zak PJ, Fischbacher U, Fehr E (2005) Oxytocin Increases Trust in Humans. Nature. 435: 673-676.
[25] Rimmele U, Hediger K, Heinrichs M, Klaver P (2009) Oxytocin Makes a Face in Memory Familiar. J. neurosci. 29: 38-42.
[26] Hurlemann R, Patin A, Onur OA, Cohen MX, Baumbartner T, Metzler S, Dziobek I, Gallinat J, Wagner M, Maier W, Kendrick KM (2010) Oxytocin Enhances Amygdala-Dependent, Socially Reinforced Learning and Emotional Empathy in Humans. J neurosci. 30: 4999-5007.
[27] Zak PJ, Stanton AA, Ahmadi S (2007) Oxytocin Increases Generosity in Humans. PLoS one. 2: e1128.
[28] Baumgartner T, Heinrichs M, Vonlanthen A, Fischbacher U, Fehr E (2008) Oxytocin Shapes the Neural Circuitry of Trust and Trust Adaptation in Humans. Neuron. 58: 639-650.
[29] Bartz JA, Zaki J, Bolger N, Ochsner KN (2011) Social Effects of Oxytocin in Humans: Context and Person Matter. Trends. cong. sci. 15: 301-309.
[30] Declerck CH, Boone C, Kiyonari T (2010) Oxytocin and Cooperation under Conditions of Uncertainty: The Modulating Role of Incentives and Social Information. Horm. behav. 57: 368-374.
[31] Shamay-Tsoory SG, Fischer M, Dvash J, Harari H, Perach-Bloom N, Levkovitz Y (2009) Intranasal Administration of Oxytocin Increases Envy and Schadenfreude (Gloating). Biol. psychiatry. 66: 864-870.
[32] Hollander E, Novotny S, Hanratty M, Yaffe R, DeCaria CM, Aronowitz BR, Mosovich S (2003) Oxytocin Infusion Reduces Repetitive Behaviors in Adults with Autistic and Asperger's Disorders. Neuropsychopharmacology, 28: 193-198.
[33] Hollander E, Bartz J, Chaplin W, Phillips A, Sumner J, Soorya L, Anagnostou E, Wasserman S (2007) Oxytocin Increases Retention of Social Cognition in Autism. Biol. psychiatry. 61: 498-503.

[34] Andari E, Duhamel JR, Zalla T, Herbrecht E, Leboyer M, Sirigu A (2010) Promoting Social Behavior with Oxytocin in High-Functioning Autism Spectrum Disorders. Proc. natl.acad. sci. u s a. 107: 4389-4394.

[35] Guastella AJ, Einfeld SL, Gray KM, Rinehart NJ, Tonge BJ, Lambert TJ, Hickie IB (2010) Intranasal Oxytocin Improves Emotion Recognition for Youth with Autism Spectrum Disorders. Biol. psychiatry. 67: 692-694.

[36] Baron-Cohen S, Wheelwright S, Hill J, Raste Y, Plumb I (2001) The "Reading the Mind in the Eyes" Test Revised Version: A Study with Normal Adults, and Adults with Asperger's Syndrome or High-Functioning Autism. J child psycho. psychiatry. 42: 241-251.

[37] Bölte S, Poustka F, Constantino JN (2008) Assessing Autistic Traits: Cross-Cultural Validation of the Social Responsiveness Scale (SRS). Autism res. 1: 354-63.

[38] Hardan AY, Fung LK, Libove RA, Obukhanych TV, Nair S, Herzenberg LA, Frazier TW, Tirouvanziam R (2012) A Randomized Controlled Pilot Trial of Oral N-Acetylcysteine in Children with Autism. Biol. psychiatry. Available: http://www.sciencedirect.com/science/article/pii/S0006322312000534. Accessed 2012 Feb 17.

[39] Geretsegger M, Holck U, Gold C (2012) Randomised Controlled Trial of Improvisational Music Therapy's Effectiveness for Children with Autism Spectrum Disorders (TIME-A): Study Protocol. BMC pediatr. 12: 2.

[40] Domes G, Heinrichs M, Michel A, Berger C, Herpertz SC (2007) Oxytocin Improves "Mind-Reading" in Humans. Biol. psychiatry. 61: 731-733.

[41] Nowicki S Jr, Duke MP (1994) Individuals Differences in the Nonverbal Communication of Affect: The Diagnostic Analysis of Nonverbal Accuracy Scale. J. nonverb. behav. 18: 9-35.

[42] Ingersoll B (2010) Broader Autism Phenotype and Nonverbal Sensitivity: Evidence for an Association in the General Population. J. autism dev. disord. 40: 590-598.

[43] Deveney CM, Brotman MA, Decker AM, Pine DS, Leibenluft E (2012) Affective Prosody Labeling in Youths with Bipolar Disorder or Severe Mood Dysregulation. J. child psychol. psychiatry. 53: 262-270.

[44] Lord C, Rutter M, Goode S, Heemsbergen J, Jordan H, Mawhood L, Schopler E (1989) Autism Diagnostic Observation Schedule: A Standardized Observation of Communicative and Social Behavior. J. autism dev. disord. 19: 185-212.

[45] Anme T, Watanabe T, Tokutake K, Tomisaki E, Mochizuki Y, Tanaka E, Wu B, Nanba M, Shinohara R, Sugisawa Y (2011) A Pilot Study of Social Competence Assessment Using Interaction Rating Scale Advanced. ISRN pediatr. 2011: 272913.

[46] McCracken JT, McGough J, Shah B, Cronin P, Hong D, Aman MG, Arnold LE, Lindsay R, Nash P, Hollway J, McDougle CJ, Posey D, Swiezy N, Kohn A, Scahill L, Martin A, Koenig K, Volkmar F, Carroll D, Lancor A, Tierney E, Ghuman J, Gonzalez NM, Grados M, Vitiello B, Ritz L, Davies M, Robinson J, McMahon D; Research Units on Pediatric Psychopharmacology Autism Network (2002) Risperidone in Children with Autism and Serious Behavioral Problems. N. engl. j. med. 347: 314-321.

[47] Liszkowski U, Carpenter M, Tomasello M (2007) Reference and Attitude in Infant Pointing. J. child lang. 34: 1-20.

[48] Werner E, Dawson G (2005) Validation of the Phenomenon of Autistic Regression Using Home Videotapes. Arch. gen. psychiatry. 62: 889-895.

[49] Koyama T, Inokuchi E, Inada N, Kuroda M, Moriwaki A, Katagiri M, Noriuchi M, Kamio Y (2010) Utility of the Japanese Version of the Checklist for Autism in Toddlers for Predicting Pervasive Developmental Disorders at Age 2. Psychiatry clin. neurosci. 64: 330-332.

[50] Williams DM, Happé F (2009) What Did I Say? Versus What Did I Think? Attributing False Beliefs to Self Amongst Children with and without Autism. J. autism dev. disord. 39: 865-873.

Section 3

Miscellaneous Issues

Chapter 6

The Effects of Some Neuropeptides on Motor Activity of Smooth Muscle Organs in Abdominal and Pelvic Cavities

Anna Tolekova, Petya Hadzhibozheva, Tsvetelin Georgiev, Stanislava Mihailova, Galina Ilieva, Maya Gulubova, Eleonora Leventieva-Necheva, Kiril Milenov and Reni Kalfin

Additional information is available at the end of the chapter

http://dx.doi.org/10.5772/48417

1. Introduction

1.1. Neuropeptides

Neuropeptides are intracellular peptides, composed of short chains of amino acids and found in brain tissue. They are often localized in axon terminals at synapses and are released as intercellular messengers that transmit information in the central nervous system, gastro-intestinal tract etc. Many are also hormones released by nonneuronal cells. Neuropeptides can be divided and grouped according their site of synthesis and secretion or their structural or functional characteristics. Currently recognized neuropeptides include all hypothalamic releasing hormones, pituitary hormones, gastro-intestinal and brain peptides, some circulating hormones, opioide peptides, neurohypophyseal hormones etc (Siegel, 2006). Some neuropeptides are secreted by the nerve terminals with conventional neurotransmitters. But which are the differences between the classical neurotransmitters and the neuropeptides? The precursors of neuropeptides have at least 90 amino acids residues - larger than the precursors of the neurotransmitters. The synthesis of neuropeptides is carried in the neuronal soma and then is transported to the axonal ends. The secretion of neuropeptides requires lower concentration of intracellular Ca^{2+} in comparison to transmitters. After secretion the neuropeptides or their precursors are reused in the synapse. The concentration of the neuropeptides in the tissue is very low and they interact with the receptors at lower concentrations than neurotransmitters. Neuropeptides appearance and secretion are very plastic (Siegel, 2006). For example in pathological conditions, the number of endocrine cells that secrete neuropeptides can not only increase but also appear unusual locations as a result of additional stimulation (Gulubova et al., 2012).

1.2. Vasopressin

Vasopressin (arginine vasopressin, AVP) is the first identified neuropeptide. AVP is a nonapeptide that is synthesized in magnocellular and parvocellular neurons, located in the paraventricular and supraoptic nuclei of the hypothalamus (Swaab et al., 1975). Most of vasopressin is released from the axonal terminals of magnocellular neurons directly iinto the bloodstream of the posterior pituitary.

The effects of AVP are mediated mainly via V1and V2 receptors.

V1 receptors are located on the vascular smooth muscle membranes. They are also found in myometrium and urinary bladder smooth muscle cell membranes. V1-receptor activation mediates vasoconstriction by receptor-coupled activation of phospholipase C and release of Ca^{2+} from intracellular stores via the phosphoinositide cascade (Thibonnier, 1992, Briley et al., 1994).

V2 renal receptors are present in the renal collecting duct system and endothelial cells. Kidney V2 receptors interact (by the G protein complex) with adenylyl cyclase to increase intracellular cyclic adenosine monophosphate (cAMP) and cause retention of water (Orloff & Handler, 1967).

V3 pituitary receptors (formerly known as V1b or AVPr1B), have central neural system effects, such as increasing adrenocorticotropic hormone production, activating different G proteins, and act via increasing intracellular cAMP (Thibonnier et al, 1997, Holmes et al, 2001, Kam et al, 2007).

The classical effects of vasopressin are mainly related to maintenance of water-electrolyte homeostasis and blood pressure. During the last years the data about the effects of this neuropeptide on brain function and behavioral reactions increase. The brain effects of vasopressin can be divided into two main types: those related to its peripheral effects such as hormone and focused on the maintenance of water balance. Others are associated with higher brain functions as learning, memory, emotion and they are independent of its hormonal effects (Frank & Landgraf, 2008). Vasopressinergic axons propelled from hypothalamus to many brain regions as hipocampus, septum, amygdala and brainstem, secrete AVP that acts as neurotransmitter. This extrahypothalamic vasopressin network is an anatomical basis of involvement of limbic-midbrain structure in processes of learning and memory. AVP facilitates consolidation and retrieval of memory (Kovacs et al., 1979)

Vasopressin participates in formation of circadian rhythms and regulation of biological clock. The suprachiasmatic nucleus (SCN) is responsible for generation of circadian rhythmicity in mammalian brain and is an obvious source for a vasopressin innervation of GABAergic neurons located in this area (Hermes et al., 2000). A significant diurnal variation in vasopressin release in the SCN was detected, with the highest levels occurring during midday and a trough around midnight (Kalsbeek et al., 1995). It was demonstrated that melatonin synthesis was stimulated after local injection in pineal gland of vasopressin. Also the night melatonin plasma concentration was increased after prolonged period of water deprivation. These results show that vasopressin can modulate melatonin synthesis in the rat pineal (Barassin et al., 2000). The suprachyasmatic nuclei, that are the main biological clock, contain vasopressinergic neurons. They demonstrate noticeable daily variation activity. In animals these vasopressin secreting neurons have very important role in the control of day/night rhythms. The reduced secretion of vasopressin in suprachyasmatic nuclei could contribute to the violation of sleep-wake rhythms during ageing and to development of depression (Kalsbeek et al., 2010).

Vasopressin takes part in the regulation of maletypical social behaviors, vocal communication, aggression, and paternal care (Goodson & Bass, 2001). There are established projections of vasopressinergic neurons from the cells of the bed nucleus of the stria terminalis to the lateral septum with higher levels of density in nonaggressive animals. These lacalizations demonstrate the significance of vasopressinergic brain network in development of aggression (Compaan, 1993).

AVP is a potent regulator of complex social maternal behaviors. The maternal cares that are vasopressin dependent were found to be independent of dam's trait anxiety. The authors suggest that manipulation of AVP system could contribute to the treatment of mothers suffering from postpartum depression (Bosch & Neumann, 2008).

Vasopressin, secreted in olfactory bulb is involved in the processing of stimuli that are important for social behaviors. In this anatomic region Tobin and coauthors (2010) have identified population of vasopressin neurons, most of which do not project outside the olfactory bulb. They discuss the importance of vasopressin secreting neurons in filtering out of the olfactory signals and in social recognition (Tobin et al., 2010).

Vasopressin and corticoliberin, secreted from parvocellular portion of paraventricular nucleus in stress condition synergistically activate ACTH-adrenal axis. Aguilera supposed that in chronic stress there is preferential activation of vasopressin rather than corticoliberin and as a consequence a feedback mechanism is disintegrated (Aguilera, 1994). In contrast Zelena et al. (2006) demonstrate that AVP does not play critical role in stimulation of hypothalamic-pituitary axis during chronic stress, but its role in acute stress is more important.

1.3. Ghrelin

Ghrelin is a multifunctional peptide hormone (28 amino acids) secreted from the cells of the diffuse neuro-endocrine system. Ghrelin-secreting cells are found from the stomach to the colon (in the oxyntic glands of the fundus and less in the small and large intestine) (Broglio et al., 2002; Lee et al., 2002; Inui et al., 2004). Ghrelin has been detected in the central nervous system, e.g. in arcuate nucleus and hypothalamus (Lu et al., 2002), in pancreas (Date et al. 2002), in some cells of the immune system (lymphocytes and monocytes) (Mager et al., 2008) and also in human ovaries and testes (García et al., 2007). There is a hypothesis that ghrelin might have not only endocrine but also autocrine and paracrine mechanism of action.

The presence of ghrelin receptor subtype GHS-R1a is detected in hypothalamus (n.arcuatus) and the pituitary gland, in multiple organs with nonendocrine and endocrine function (heart, lung, liver, kidney, pancreas, stomach, small and large intestines, adipose tissue, immune cells, gonads, thyroid gland, adrenal gland) (Broglio et al., 2003; Inui et al., 2004; Van Der Lely et al., 2004) and in gastrointestinal vasculature (Mladenov et al., 2006). They are also expressed by lumbosacral autonomic preganglionic neurons of the micturition reflex pathways (Ferens et al., 2010)

The activation of the receptor causes the stimulation of the G-protein subunit Gα11. This leads to the activation of intracellular signaling cascades via the phospholipase C (PLC) (Vartiainen, 2009).

The principal physiological action of ghrelin is the stimulation of secretion of growth hormone. Therefore ghrelin is a hormone with anabolic effect. It participates in the regulation of metabolism, energy homeostasis and feeding behaviors which are mediated via a complex neuroendocrine network (Van Der Lely et al., 2004). Ghrelin increases appetite and food intake and decreases fat utilisation as a metabolic fuel and increases fat storage in the adipose tissue. Ghrelin modulates gastic motility and emptying and gastric acid secretion and stimulates ileum peristalsis, most of these effects being vagally mediated (Ghigo et al., 2005). It induces fasted motor activity in the duodenum (Fujino et al., 2003). Ghrelin activity is mediated via enteric nervous system (Tack et al., 2006).

Ghrelin and its receptors are present not only in the peripheral tissues but also in the central nervous system (Kang et al., 2011). Ghrelin functions as a peripheral hormone that is released mainly from the stomach and affects the hypothalamus, but also as a neuropeptide in hypothalamus (Kojima and Kangawa, 2005). Like other neuropeptides, Ghrelin is widely distributed in the brain in key areas of emotional regulation, and plays role as modulators of behavioural states (Kang et al., 2011). Ghrelin plays an important role in the regulation of energy balance by regulating food intake, body weight, glucose homeostasis and feeding behaviour which are mediated by a complex neuroendocrine network (Kalra et al., 1999; Van Der Lely et al., 2004). The regulation of energy balance is related to somatic growth and instinctive behaviour, including feeding, reproduction and emotion, and is a complex phenomenon involving interaction of the central and peripheral nervous systems, neuroendocrine system and gastrointestinal system (Matsuda et al., 2011). Ghrelin induces in the brain an orexigenic effect, modifies locomotor activity and also is involved in the control of psychophysiological functions and regulation of metabolism (Kang et al., 2011). The hypothalamic region of the brain plays very important role in the regulation of feeding and neuroendocrine functions (Kalra et al., 1999). Many types of neurons in the hypothalamus and related regions express ghrelin and some neuropeptides, such as, orexin, NPY, agouti-related peptide (AGRP), melanin-concentrating hormone (MCH) and other, which are implicated in the regulation of feeding behaviour and also in energy homeostasis in mammals (Eva et al., 2006; Kalra et al., 1999; Pickar et al., 1993). Ghrelin increases orexigenic effect and food intake but decreases energy expenditure thus inducing weight gain. (Kojima & Kangawa, 2005; Van Der Lely et al., 2004). Ghrelin exerts its central orexigenic effect through activation of hypothalamic neurons in the arcuate nucleus, important area involved in the regulation of energy balance and in addition it stimulates the neurons of other areas of the central nervous system, for example nucleus paraventricularis, dorsomedial parts of hypothalamus, and areas in the brain stem nucleus tractus solitarius and the area postrema, which all take part in the modulation of appetite control (Lim et al., 2010; Vartiainen, 2009). Ghrelin-secreting hypothalamic neurons send efferent fibers onto key circuits involved in the central regulation of energy homeostasis. They balance the activity of orexigenic neuropeptide Y/agouti-related peptide neurons in the arcuate nucleus and the activity of anorexigenic pro-opiomelanocortin (POMC) neurons that secrete alpha melanocyte stimulating hormone (α-MSH) and thus modulate the resultant effect (Van Der Lely et al., 2004).

Several new intracellular targets/mediators of the appetite-inducing effect of ghrelin in the hypothalamus have recently been identified, including the AMP-activated protein kinase, its upstream kinase calmodulin kinase kinase 2, components of the fatty acid pathway and the uncoupling protein 2 (Lim et al., 2010).

Recently, it has been demonstrated that ghrelin plays an important role in the regulation of central and peripheral lipid metabolism through specific control of hypothalamic AMP-activated protein kinase (AMPK), a critical metabolic regulator of both cellular and whole-body energy homeostasis (Kola et al., 2005).

Centrally administered ghrelin has various effects such as arousal, increasing gastric acid secretion and gastrointestinal motility, inhibition of water intake and release of some hormones from the pituitary, mainly growth hormone (Hashimoto et al., 2011).

Ghrelin may be synthesized in the hypothalamus. Ghrelin have hypothalamic actions on growth hormone-releasing hormone neurons (Sun et al., 2007). Ghrelin acts centrally to exert a global stimulatory effect on the hypothalamo-pituitary-adrenal axis. Ghrelin increases absolute whole adrenal gland weight and whole adrenal gland volume and elevates blood concentrations of ACTH, aldosterone and corticosterone (Milosević VLj et al., 2010). Ghrelin may function as a metabolic modulator of the gonadotropic axis, with inhibitory effects in line with its role as signal of energy deficit. These effects likely include inhibition of luteinizing hormone secretion, as well as partial suppression of normal puberty onset (Tena-Sempere, 2008).

Ghrelin-immunoreactive neurons are present in the paraventricular, dorsomedial, ventromedial and arcuate nuclei, areas important for circadian output. Contrary to the effects of ghrelin on appetite, growth hormone release and the sleep–wake cycle, little is known about the effects of ghrelin on circadian rhythms (Yannielli et al., 2007).

Central ghrelin is also a gastroprotective factor in gastric mucosa. The gastric protection elicited by central ghrelin requires integrity of capsaicin-sensitive sensory neurons, which play an important role in gastric cytoprotection. Growing evidence indicates that the mechanisms triggered by peptides to increase resistance of the gastric mucosa involve changes in the release of gastric protective factors. Endogenous prostaglandins are involved in ghrelin gastroprotection (Sibilia et al., 2008).

The short-term activation of AMPK in turn results in decreased hypothalamic levels of malonyl-CoA and increased carnitine palmitoyltransferase 1 (CPT1) activity. Ghrelin deficiency induces reductions in both de novo lipogenesis and beta-oxidation pathways in the hypothalamus. There are reductions in fatty acid synthase (FAS) mRNA expression both in the ventromedial nucleus of the hypothalamus and whole hypothalamus, as well as in FAS protein and activity. CPT1 activity is also reduced. Chronic ghrelin treatment does not promote AMPK-induced changes in the overall fluxes of hypothalamic fatty acid metabolism in normal rats and this effect is independent of ghrelin status. In addition, ghrelin plays a dual time-dependent role in modulating hypothalamic lipid metabolism. (Diéguez C et al., 2010; Sangiao-Alvarellos et al., 2010)

A reciprocal relationship exists between ghrelin and insulin, suggesting that ghrelin regulates glucose homeostasis (Sun et al., 2007).

1.4. Angiotensin II

The octapeptide Angiotensin II (Ang II) is the main effector of the renin-angiotensin system (RAS). Ang II is generated in circulation or locally in tissues in the kidney, blood vessels, heart, and brain and etc.

The signal transduction mechanism for AT1 receptors is well known. AT1 receptors are distributed in adult tissues including blood vessel, heart, kidney, adrenal gland, liver, brain, and lung. These receptors activate phospholipase A2, phospholipase C, phospholipase D and L-type Ca^{2+} channels and inhibiting the adenylyl cyclase (Shokei & Hiroshi, 2011).

AT2 receptors are ubiquitously expressed in developing fetal tissues, suggesting a possible role of these receptors in fetal development and organ morphogenesis. AT2 receptors expression rapidly decreases after birth, and in the adult. Expression of these receptors are limited mainly to the uterus, ovary, certain brain nuclei, heart, and adrenal medulla. In various cell lines, AT2 receptors activated protein tyrosine phosphatase was shown to inhibit cell growth or induce programmed cell death (apoptosis) (Kim and Awao, 2011).

Ang II has a multifunctional role. It is general regulator of salt and water metabolism, thirst, sympathetic outflow and vascular smooth muscle cell tone. As a result Ang II acts as a principal controller of long term regulation of blood pressure (Robertson, 2005; Watanabe et al., 2005). Later, Ang II was found to exert long-term effects on tissue structure, including cardiac hypertrophy, vascular remodeling, and renal fibrosis (Watanabe et al., 2005).

The key effector of peripheral renin-angiotensin system (RAS) - Ang II in circulation does not cross blood-brain barrier. Therefore it interacts on brain regions that lack the blood-brain barrier as circumventricular areas, organum vasculosum laminae terminalis, where Ang II stimulates salt appetite, thirst and vasopressin secretion (Fitts et al., 2000). Also, it influences neuronal activity in area postrema and takes part in central regulation of blood pressure (Otsuka et al., 1986).

Many immunohistochemical studies demonstrate the distribution of all components of RAS - angiotensinogen, Ang I, Ang II and renin in several brain regions of rats. Immunoreactivity for Ang II was detected in neurons and vessels in the brainstem, cerebellum, hypothalamus, basal ganglia, thalamus and cortex while for angiotensinogen and Ang I were found in neurons of the hypothalamic nuclei in rats (McKinley et al., 2003; Von Bohlen et al., 2006). AT1 receptor binding sites with higher density were localized in the lamina terminalis, hypothalamic paraventricular nucleus and the nucleus tractus solitaries, lamina terminalis and the subfornical organ. The median preoptic nucleus also contains membranes rich in AT1 receptors. All regions that are included in the regulation of cardiovascular functions as caudal ventrolateral medulla, and the midline raphe, also have AT1receptors (Allen et al., 1999; Lenkei et al., 1997). In the midbrain -in the lateral parabrachial nucleus, substantia nigra and periaqueductal gray AT1 receptors are presented from moderate to high densities (Lenkei et al., 1997). These localizations of RAS brain components show that Ang II is involved in the regulations of thirst, drinking, facilitating vasopressor effects and secretion of vasopressin, adrenocorticotrophic and luteinizing hormones. Ang II also stimulates secretion of neurotransmitters such as noradrenaline and 5-hydroxytryptamine (5-HT) and inhibits acetylcholine release. The brain RAS appears to be also an important modulator of the blood pressure circadian rhythm and it influences renal renin release.

Recent findings demonstrate that central effects of Ang II contribute to facilitated learning and enhance associative memory and learning possibly with differential effects on acquisition, storage and recall. Brain RAS is involved in the development of affective disorders and Ang II has a modulating effect of on anxiety (Georgiev & Yonkov, 1985).

RAS receptors alterations have been found in some neurodegenerative disorders - Parkinson's and Huntington's disease (Ge & Barnes, 1996). The number of AT1 receptors in caudate nucleus, putamen and substantia nigra was significantly decreased in Parkinson's disease patients in comparison to controls. In Huntington's disease patients, AT1receptors was found to be slightly decreased in putamen (Ge & Barnes, 1996). AT2 receptors that are localized in caudate nucleus was decreased in Parkinson's and increased in Huntington's disease patients. The receptor alterations were considerable; therefore the authors have concluded that brain RAS seems to decisively contribute to the pathology of the dopaminergic nigrostriatal pathway in these patients and may be a novel therapeutic target for neurodegenerative disorders (Savaskan, 2005).

1.5. Cholecystokinin

In 1928 Ivy and Oldberg extracted from dog duodenal mucosis a substance which injected intravenously contracted the gallbladder. The authors named this substance cholecystokinin (CCK). Later, Harper & Raper (1943) found a compound in this extract that stimulated the pancreatic secretion and called it pancreozymin. Purifying both hormones and determing their amino-acid sequention, Mutt (1980) proved them to be the same linear polypeptide, containing 33 amino-acid residues, and proposed the hybrid name "cholecystokinin-pancreozymin". Different CCK forms have been shown to exist: CCK-58, CCK-39, CCK-33, CCK-27, CCK-12, CCK-8, CCK-4, all of them containing a bioactive C-terminal. CCK-58 and CCK-39 are precursors of CCK-33 and by the degradation of the latter the shorter forms are obtained. Cholecystokinin octapeptide (CCK-8) is the most active one and is most widely spread in the gastro-intestinal tract and in the central nervous system. A cholecystokinin analogue, named caerulein, has been isolated from the skin of the frog *Hyla caerulea*.

CCK and gastrin possess identical 5 aminoacids at their C-terminals that are the biologically active part of both hormones. The dissimilarities in their potency and physiological activity are determined by the different positions of the *Tyr*-residue in the molecules of both peptides. When the *Tyr*-residue is in the 6th position, the peptide (gastrin) strongly potentiates the gastric secretion, its stimulating effect on the gallbladder contractions and pancreating secretion being much weaker. With the *Tyr*-residue in the 7th position, CCK markedly enhances the gallbladder motility and the pancreatic secretion.

Immunohistochemical studies have shown that CCK is synthesized in the mucosal endocrine cells type I and type K of the small intestine, and in the endocrine cells type A of the pancreas. CCK-immunoreactivity has been also identified in the vagus nerve. Cholecystokinin is so called "brain-gut" neuropeptide – it is also produced by enteric neurons, and is widely and abundantly distributed in the brain.

The food intake in the small intestine is the main physiological stimulus for the CCK release – masts, proteins and aminoacids are the most powerful stimulants among the foods. The plasma CCK concentration increases from 1-2 pmol/l to 6-8 pmol/l after feeding (Cantor, 1986). Cholecystokinin plays a key role in facilitating digestion within the small intestine – this peptide stimulates delivery into the small intestine of digestive enzymes from the pancreas and bile from the gallbladder. Recently it was shown that CCK-8 can reduce food intake by capsaicin-insensitive, nonvagal mechanisms (Zhang & Ritter, 2012).

Mechanisms of secretion of cholecystokinin group peptides into the gastro-intestinal tract are as follows: a) Endocrine mechanism – the peptide is released by the endocrine cell in a blood vessel and is afterwards transported by the circulation to the effector cell; b) Paracrine mechanism – the peptide is released by the endocrine cell in the intracellular space, reaching afterwards the effector cell by diffusion; c) Neurotransmitter mechanism – the peptide is released by the nerve terminal in the synaptic cleft and affects afterwards the activity of the effector neuron; d) Neuroendocrine mechanism – the peptide is released by the neuron in a blood vessel.

The peptide hormone CCK realizes its effects via binding to specific receptors localized on the cell membranes of the target organs. Two types of cholecystokinin receptors have been characterized so far: CCK_A and CCK_B which are approximately 50 % homologous (Dufresne et al., 2006).

CCK_A (gastro-intestinal) receptors. They prevail in the peripheral target organs (pancreas, gallbladder, small intestine), as well as in the vagus nerve afferent fibres, mediating the pancreatic enzyme secretion and the gallbladder and ileum motility (Crawley & Corwin, 1994; Xu et al., 2008). CCK_A-receptors have also been identified in some brain regions where they take part in the modulation of dopaminergic neurotransmission, and in the regulation of food behavior - satiety effect (Lieverse et al., 1995).

CCK_B (brain) receptors. They have been identified in various brain structures, as their number is largest in the cortex, hippocampus and limbic structures (Hokfelt et al., 1985). CCK_B receptors, similar or identical to the peripheral gastrin receptors, have been demonstrated in peripheral organs, too.

Cholecystokinin is a major peptide hormone in the gut and a major peptide transmitter in the brain. Its synthesis requires endoproteolytic cleavage of proCCK at several mono- and dibasic sites by prohormone convertases. On one hand cholecystokinin is a classical gut hormone and a growth factor for the pancreas. On the other, the CCK gene is expressed also in large quantities in cerebral and peripheral neurons from where CCK peptides are released as potent neurotransmitters and modulators. Accordingly, cerebral CCK defects have been associated with major neuropsychiatric diseases such as anxiety, schizophrenia and satiety disorders (Crawley & Corwin, 1994; Liddle, 1997).

CCK is also a key component of the aggression facilitating circuitry in the brain (Luo et al., 1998), and it is released during inter-male fighting (Becker et al., 2001). In addition to its many aversive motivational/emotional effects, CCK also plays a role in more positively valenced motivational states, such as mating (Dornan & Malsbury, 1989; Markowski & Hull, 1995), drug addiction (Crespi, 2000) and brain reward processes (Degen et al., 2001, Josselyn, 1996).

It was demonstrated that CCK is colocalized with dopamine in ventral striatal dopamine neurons (Hokfelt et al., 1980). Consistent with the neuronal colocalization and extensive overlap of expression between CCK and the dopaminergic system, CCK peptides have significant effects on dopamine mediated behaviors. Administration of CCK peptides exhibit many of the behavioral characteristics of antipsychotics including inhibition of conditioned avoidance responding (Cohen et al., 1982), inhibition of apomorphine-induced stereotypic behavior (Zetler, 1983), and inhibitionof amphetamine-induced hyperlocomotion (Schneider et al., 1983). Microinjection of CCK into the anterior nucleus accumbens inhibits dopamine release, inhibits dopamine-mediated behaviors and is blocked by a CCK_A antagonist whereas injection into the posterior nucleus accumbens has the opposite effects and these effects are mediated by CCK_B receptors (Vaccarino & Rankin, 1989, Crawley, 1992). Thus, it appears that different CCK-based circuitries in the brain can facilitate both negative and positive emotional processes. It is also interesting to note that selective CCK_B agonists that cross the blood brain barrier such as pentagastrin and CCK-4 are used to induce panic attacks in clinical studies. Consequently, a CCK agonist for schizophrenia would need to be either nonselective or CCK_A selective.

CCK was the first gut hormone discovered to have anoretic effects. Its actions include inhibition of food intake, delayed gastric emptying, stimulation of pancreatic enzyme secretion, and stimulation of gall bladder contraction. These effects are mediated via binding to CCK receptors on the vagus nerve. CCK administration to humans and animals inhibits food intake by reducing meal size and duration. However, at high dose nausea and taste aversion have been detected making CCK an unlikely candidate for an anti-obesity treatment.

2. Materials and methods

Wistar rats of both sexes weighting 200–250 g were used. The experiment was carried out in accordance with the national regulations and DIRECTIVE 2010/63/EU of the European Parliament and of the Council of 22 September 2010 concerning the protection of animals used for scientific and experimental purposes. The animals were anesthetized with Nembutal 50 mg/kg intraperitoneally and exsanguinated. Abdominal cavity was opened and longitudinal strips from different parts of gastro-intestinal tract, urinary bladder and uterus horn were dissected out. The isolated organs were transferred immediately in cold Krebs solution 3 °C), containing following composition in mM): NaCl—118.0, KCl—4.74, $NaHCO_3$—25.0, $MgSO_4$—1.2, $CaCl_2$—2.0, KH_2PO_4—1.2 and glucose 11.0.

Longitudinal strips approximately 2 mm wide, 0.5 mm thick and 8 mm long) were dissected following the direction of the muscle bundles. The two ends of each strip were tied with silk ligatures. The distal end was connected to the organ holder; the proximal end was stretched and attached to a mechano-electrical transducer FSG-01 (Experimetria, Ltd., Hungary) via a hook. The preparations were mounted in organ baths TSZ-04/01, containing Krebs solution, pH 7.4, continuously bubbled with Carbogen (95% O_2, 5% CO_2). The organ baths were mounted in parallel above an enclosed water bath, maintaining the solution temperature at 37 °C. Each smooth muscle strip was initially stretched to a tension of 1.0 g followed by 90 minutes of equilibration. During this period, the smooth muscle strips were replenished with fresh Krebs solution at 15-th min, 60-th min and 75-th min.

After initial period of adaptation, they were treated with the solution of different neuropeptides, and the obtained responses were registered.

The phasic contractions of the smooth muscles before application of neuropeptide and the changes of motor activity, expressed as tonic contractions, relaxations or lack of reaction after treatment were recorded. The contractile activity signals were transduced by mechanical-force sensor, amplified, digitized and recorded using ISOSYS ADVANCED digital acquisition software, produced by Experimetria Ltd., Hungary.

Chemicals and drugs

Ang II (Sigma-Aldrich), vasopressin (Sigma-Aldrich), ghrelin (PolyPeptide Group) synthetic octapeptide of cholecystokinin (Squibb, USA), acetylcholine chloride (Sigma-Aldrich), hexamethonium chloride (Sigma-Aldrich) were solubilized in bidistillated water. All reagents for the preparation of Krebs solution were purchased from Sigma-Aldrich.

Data analysis and statistic processing

The recorded force-vs.-time curves permit determination of amplitudes and integrated force of contraction, the latter represented by the area under the curve (AUC), as well as defining of time parameters. Data acquisition and the initial conversion of the experimental data for the later analysis was performed with KORELIA – Processing software (Yankov, 2010). For later analysis, evaluation and identification was used KORELIA-Dynamics program. (Yankov, 2006; Yankov, 2011).

Following time parameters were examined Figure 1:

- T_{hc} *(s)* – first half contraction time - time interval between the start of the smooth muscle contraction (SMC) and half-contraction moment ($T_{hc} = t_{hc} - t_0$);

- $T_{(c-hc)}$ *(s)* – second half contraction time - - time interval between the end of Thc and maximum peak of the SMC ($T_{(c-hc)} = t_{peak}-t_{hc}$)
- T_c *(s)* – contraction time - time interval between the start of the SMC and the moment of the maximum peak ($T_c = t_{peak} - t_0$);
- T_{hr} *(s)* – half-relaxation time: time interval between the moment of the maximum peak t_{peak} and the moment when the curve decreases to $F_{max}/2$ ($T_{hr} = t_{hr} - t_{peak}$);
- T_{chr} *(s)* – contraction plus half-relaxation time: time between the start of the SMC and t_{hr} ($T_{chr} = t_{hr} – t_0$).

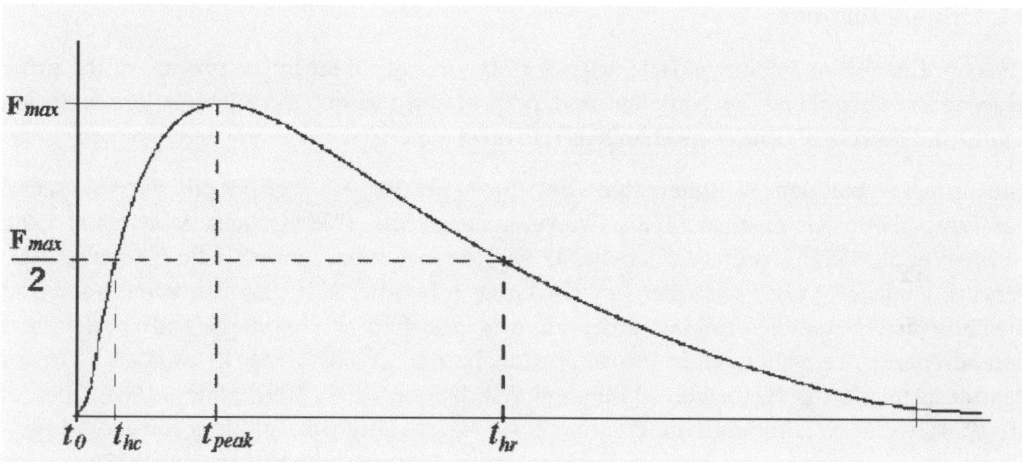

Figure 1. Smooth muscle contraction (SMC) - graph and parameters. Fmax – maximal force of the SMC; Fmax/2 – half of maximal force of the SMC; t_0 – start of SMC. t 0 = 0; t_{hc} – half-contraction moment; t_{peak} – the moment of the maximum peak Fmax; t_{hr} – the moment when the curve decreases to Fmax/2.

The duration of the tonic contraction was defined from the beginning of the contraction, until the amplitude fell to 50%.

For a more correct and acurate comparison between the parts of the gastrointestinal tract was performed normalization of the different intervals as a relative part of total length of the process Txn=Tx/chr). As a result the following normalized parameters were obtained: T_{hcn}, T_{cn}, $T_{(c-hc)n}$, T_{hrn}.

The gall bladder pressure *in vivo* was recorded in six conscious dogs weighing 18 to 20 kg. The animals were starved for 18 hours and were then anesthetized with chloralose (90 mg/kg i.v.). Laparotomy was performed through upper midline abdominal incision. Gall bladder bile was aspirated with a syringe. The bile volume was between 30 and 40 ml. A small balloon mounted on the top of a polyethylene catheter was introduced into the gall bladder. Experiments were started four weeks after surgery and were carried out twice a week at of at least two-day intervals. The dogs were deprived of food, but were given water *ad libitum* for 18 hours before each trial. The balloon was filled with 1 ml distilled water and connected through a catheter to a pressure transducer. The changes in gall bladder pressure were measured in mmHg. The first 40-min records were used as controls. Cholecystokinin octapeptide was then injected i.v. at increasing doses every 30 min. Atropine or hexamethonium was administered before cholecystokinin.

Obtained data were processed by the statistical program Statistica 6.1, StaSoft, Inc. and presented as mean ± standard error. A P-value less than or equal to 0.05 was considered to be statistically significant.

3. Results and discussions

3.1. Urinary bladder

The coordination of smooth muscle activity of the urinary tract in the process of the urine evacuation is regulated by complex, and not yet fully understood interactions between neural and hormonal control mechanisms (Dixon et al., 1997).

The urinary bladder is innervated by three groups of peripheral nerves: sacral parasympathetic (Helm et al., 1982; Crowe & Burnstock, 1989; Gabella & Uvelius, 1990; Lasanen et al., 1992; Uvelius & Gabella, 1998), thoracolumbar sympathetic (Downie, 1981; Feher & Vajda, 1981) and sacral sensory (De Groat & Booth, 1993). According to the secreted mediator in the neural terminals innervation is classified as cholinergic, adrenergic, and non-adrenergic, non-cholinergic (NANC) (Callahan & Creed, 1986). In humans detrusor neurotransmission is exclusively cholinergic (Andersson et al., 1982; Sibley, 1984; Chen et al., 1994), while its adrenergic innervation is sparse, nonuniform, and it is considered non-essential for micturition function (de Groat & Booth, 1984; Janig & McLachlan, 1987).

A lot of different neuropeptides have been found to be synthesized, stored and released from organs in the lower urinary tract (LUT). Some of them are secreted from the peripheral neural terminals of the autonomic nervous system – vasoactive intestinal peptide (VIP), tachykinins (substance P), neuropeptide Y, calcitonin gene-related peptide, neurokinin A. Others which act by para- and autocrine mechanisms as angiotensin II are locally synthesized. The exact function of many of these peptides has not been fully established, however they may play role in a sensory and efferent innervation (de Groat & Kawatani, 1985; Burnstock, 1990; Maggi, 1991) or serve as neuromodulators in the ganglia or at the neuromuscular junctions. Their actions have been thought to include mediation of the micturition reflex activation, smooth muscle contraction, potentiation of efferent neurotransmission and changes in vascular tone and permeability (Maggi, 1991, 1995; Hernandez et al., 2006).

A few hormones with systemic circulation – vasopressin, oxytocin, are influencing bladder function (Uvelius B. et al., 1990; Romine & Anderson, 1985). These also include a newly discovered peptide ghrelin, which is secreted from the gastrointestinal tract, and stimulates contractions of smooth muscles of blood vessels and gastro-intestinal tract (Tack et al., 2006; Wiley & Davenport, 2002)

Angiotensin II and urinary bladder

There is insufficient information on the effect of Ang II on non-cardiovascular organ smooth muscles (Touyz & Berry, 2002). The interactions of the Ang II with the urinary bladder are of particular interest regarding the genesis and treatment of the disorders of the micturition. The physiological effects of Ang II on the function of the urinary bladder and the transduction mechanisms which mediate it have not been fully elucidated. Ang II and its precursor Ang I cause dose-dependent contractions of muscle strips from rat urinary bladder (Andersson et al., 1992). According to experimental data of Anderson and co-authors Ang II acts as a modulator in neurotransmission in the urinary bladder (Andersson & Arner, 2004). There are research data confirming that Ang II carries out its physiological effects by binding to membrane AT1 receptors (Tanabe et al.,1993), whose number on the surface of detrusor smooth muscle cells is regulated by the dietary content of sodium and potassium and the age of experimental animals (Weaver-Osterholtz et al., 1996; Szigeti et al., 2005). AT1 receptors activate PLC, dihydropyridine-sensitive Ca^{2+}-channels and inhibit adenylilcyclase, thus reducing intracellular cAMP concentration (Chiu et al., 1994).

Our experiments show that the administration of Ang II solution to the smooth muscle stirps induce tonic contractions, in confirmation of the findings from other researchers concerning its effect on urinary bladder contractile activity. The increased amplitude of contraction following the administration of Ang II in the presence of increased extracellular Ca^{2+} provided evidence of additive synergism (Hadzhibozheva et al., 2009; Tolekova et al., 2010). The blockade of AngII-induced tonic contraction after the administration of blockers of T-type Ca^{2+} -channels unequivocally showed the role of transmembrane Ca^{2+} -influx in the initiation of smooth muscle contraction (Ilieva et al., 2008). The Ang II bindings to its membrane receptors, leads to activation of phospholipase C, which results in formation of inositol triphosphate, which triggers release of Ca^{2+} from sarcoplasmatic reticulum (SR). It's also well known that Ang II causes calcium-induced calcium release in smooth-muscle cells. Angiotensin II causes depolarization and opening of VDCC, providing additional Ca^{2+} influx from the extracellular fluid (Seki et al., 1999). When moving inside the cell, Ca^{2+} binds to ryanodine receptors and triggers supplementary Ca^{2+} release from SR stores (Berridge, 2008). In the experiment we applied specific inhibitor to this particular calcium-induced Ca^{2+} release mechanism. The resulting lack of tonic contraction suggested that this signaling pathway, leading to intracellular calcium increase is of greater importance for the development of detrusor muscle contraction than the inositol triphosphate pathway. Our experimental data also showed that the increase of calcium in extracellular fluid produced additive synergistic effect on Ang II-mediated contraction of detrusor smooth muscle strips.

The circulating AngII is formed in blood under influence of angiotensin–converting enzyme (ACE). During the last decade a lot of new facts that significantly broaden our knowledge of the RAS have been accumulated. Local tissue RAS was found in the blood vessels, heart, kidneys, small intestines, pancreatic tissue, liver, ovarics and brain (Paul at al., 2006). Other enzymes involved in RAS and physiologicaly active metabolites of Ang I and Ang II were also found (Waldeck et al., 1997; Miyazaki & Takai, 2006).

A lot of recent studies have shown that Ang II acts as a cytokine and growth-like factor. (Kim & Iwao, 2000; Touyz & Berry, 2002). It regulates the smooth muscle mass in the bladder wall in normal and pathological conditions. Chronic bladder outlet obstruction causes changes in smooth muscle mass and connective tissue both in humans' disease and under experimental conditions in rats (Yamada et al., 2009). The application of ACE blocking substances significantly reduce the quantity of the newly synthesized collagen in the bladder, which is an indirect indicator of the effects of the local RAS on developing pathologic hypertrophic changes in the bladder. Phull and coauthors (2007) showed that applying angiotensin receptor anatagonists, reduced urethral resistance on rat models with stress urinary incontinence.

The all main components of RAS – Ang I, Ang II and ACE are found inside bladder tissues (Weaver-Osterholtz et al., 1996). Tissue levels of Ang I and Ang II were higher than circulating levels, which confirms the existence of local synthesis in the urinary bladder, despite the lower measured activity of the angiotensin-converting enzyme, insitu is relatively This fact supports the hypothesis of auto- and paracrine actions of Ang II. It has been shown that Ang I also causes contraction of smooth muscle cells of the bladder, through the interaction with AT1 receptors.

Ang II -mediated contraction is not completely blocked after administration of ACE inhibitor (Lindberg et al., 1994). These facts indicate the existence of alternative pathways for the synthesis of Ang II. Urata and co-authors show that in the heart of the main enzyme converting Ang I to Ang II is a serine protease human himase (Urata et al., 1990). Andersson and co-authors found that application of enalaprilat not fully block contraction of urinary bladder detrusor stripts induced by Ang I (Andersson et al., 1992). This means that the remaining contractile effect is due to separate mechanism of Ang II formation.

Vasopressin

Besides its vasoconstrictor activity, AVP is involved in the modulation of the intrinsic smooth muscle activity of the urinary system. Vargiu and coauthors demonstrate that AVP increases the contractile activity of upper urinary tract that is most pronounced in small calices, which are the main pacemaker of the urinary tract and is mediated by V1 receptors (Vargiu et al., 2004). It remains unaffected by the blockade of sodium channels with tetrodotoxin. However, the application of nifedipine and L-type calcium channels blockers reduced spontaneous and AVP-induced activity of smooth muscles of the upper urinary tract (Vargiu et al., 2004). This demonstrates the importance of transmembrane calcium influx for the contractile activity of smooth muscle of the lower urinary tract.

There is a data that shows the presence of V1-receptors in smooth muscle of the urinary bladder, who's binding to AVP leads to activation of the inositol-triphosphate (IP_3) pathway, similarly to binding to Ang II (Crankshaw, 1989; Dehpour et al., 1997). It was found that the removal of extracellular calcium prevents the effects of AVP, suggesting it possible involvement in the activation process (Crankshaw, 1989). In our experiments AVP application to the bladder detrusor smooth muscle strips stimulates powerful tonic contractions. This result supports currently available information on this issue (Uvelius et al., 1990).

Comparison of the effects of Ang II and AVP on contractile activity

Ang II and AVP, accomplish their effects through the formation of the second messenger IP_3. The comparison of the independent effects of Ang II and AVP on urinary bladder strips shows contractions with approximately equal amplitude, but with integrated muscle force significantly increased after the application of AVP (Figure 2, Table 1) (Tolekova et al., 2010).

	Fmax.g)	AUCgs)	T_{hc} s)	$T_{c-hc)}$	T_c s)	T_{hr} s)	T_{chr}s)
AVP	1,55±0,16	761,29±113,3	28±4	99,6±15	127,4±18	255,3±35	382,7±43
Ang II	1,73±0,26	115,13±20,7	12,6±1,6	19,7±5	32,3±3,3	61,5±13,6	93,7±13,3

Table 1. Force and time-parametes means±SE) of Ang II- and AVP-induced contractions.

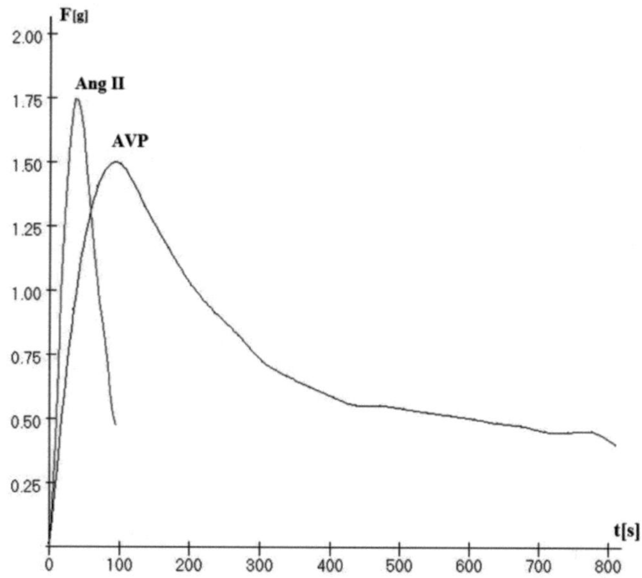

Figure 2. Angiotensin II- and AVP – induced contractions after processing of signals with specialized software.

For detailed study and comparison of the tonic contractions under the influence of the two peptides, we are using time parameters, described in Yankov (2011) (Figure 1, Table 1), generated after signal processing with specialized software (Yankov, 2010). The similar parameters were used for investigation of the contractions of the skeletal muscles (Raikova & Aladjov, 2004). Our research results show that Ang II causes contractions with a shorter duration (shorter time for reaching Fmax/2 and Fmax). The AVP-induced response reaches significant AUC value at the expense of the lower rate of increased and decreased contractile activity (longer duration of Thr and Tchr). The greater length of AVP contraction time is mainly due to longer $T_{(c-hc)}$ period. It is particularly interesting that despite acting through the same transduction pathways, Ang II and AVP cause tonic contractions with different measured force. We assume that this difference, especially the higher speed of relaxation, might be related to the specific Ang II metabolism in bladder cells. Production of Ang III and Ang 1-7 may be a cause of the faster rate of relaxation (Varagic et al., 2008). The interactions of the two peptides – Ang II and AVP with the ion channels of the smooth muscle membrane may contribute additionally to the differences in the computed parameters and shape of the contraction graphic. There are existing data about the effect of AVP on the potassium channels of brain cells after fluid percussion brain injury indicating that AVP inhibited activity of the KATP and KCa channels (Armstead, 2001). It is known that the urinary bladder smooth muscle cells have a number of potassium channels, including ATP-dependent K channels and Ca^{2+}-dependent K channels (Petkov et al., 2001). Interaction with those channels could be a possible explanation for the prolonged duration of AVP action on smooth muscle contractions.

On the other hand, Ang II stimulates the activity of L/T-type voltage dependent calcium channels in vascular smooth muscle cells (Lu et al., 1996). We can suggest that in the smooth muscle cells of the rat bladder a similar effect takes place.

Role of extracellular calcium for Ang II- and AVP-mediated contractions of smooth muscle cells

The increase of concentration of the extracellular Ca^{2+} exerts a synergistic effect on Ang II- and AVP-mediated contractions. The raise of the amplitude of contraction is a consequence of increased transmembrane calcium influx due to the higher electrochemical gradient. As a result the intracellular calcium concentration is maintained at the higher level than the level of the resting state. There is evidence that this pattern of variations in calcium concentration contributes to the development of the mechanism of "locking" of the smooth muscle cells (Tanaka et al., 2008). We suppose that the above mentioned significant difference in AUC is due to the manifestation of this mechanism (Tolekova et al., 2010).

Ghrelin

The endocrine effects of the peptide ghrelin on various organs and systems are not well examined; however it is known that it stimulates the motility of digestive tract (Tack et al., 2006). On the vascular smooth muscle it exercises a dilatatory influence which is comparable to that caused by adrenomeduline (Wiley & Davenport, 2002). Binding of ghrelin to the its membrane receptors in some tissues triggers signal transduction mechanism via Gq protein and results in activation of PLC and release of IP_3 and Ca^{2+} (Davenport et al., 2005). There are no data in the literature regarding the effects of ghrelin on urinary bladder smooth muscle. The presence of ghrelin receptors on the membranes of detrusor smooth muscle cells is not proven yet. Therefore it is interesting to investigate whether and how ghrelin affects the bladder detrusor and if so by which signal transduction mechanism. Moreover, there is not existing published comparison between the effects of AVP and Ang II on detrusor contractile activity as well as effects of calcium and ghrelin on the smooth-muscle contractions mediated by these peptides.

Does Ghrelin have an effect on a urinary bladder?

The receptors for ghrelin described in the literature mediate their activity with activation of PLC and subsequent increase in concentration of intracellular calcium (Davenport et al., 2005). Therefore, the application of ghrelin on muscle strips of urinary bladder would lead to the occurrence of tonic contractions. During the experiments we found no statistically significant changes in contractile activity after application of ghrelin as compared to the spontaneous activity. The effects of ghrelin are displayed only when it is applied in combination with other peptides – Ang II or AVP. In combination with Ang II, ghrelin reduces its contractile effect on the bladder (Ilieva et al., 2008, a). The combination of ghrelin with AVP leads to similar yet significantly less manifested decrease, especially in the AUC.

Based on these results we can assume that the urinary bladder possesses receptors for ghrelin, different from those in the digestive tract, with respect to the intracellular signaling mechanism to which they are coupled. The significant reduction in the amplitude of Ang II-induced contraction as well as the partial reduction of AVP-provoked contraction after ghrelin application could be explained by the interaction between signal transduction pathways by which the both peptides act. To our knowledge, this is the first *in vitro* study demonstrated the inhibitory effect of ghrelin on bladder motor activity. Our results were confirmed by Matsuda et coauthors (2011). They showed in experiments in vivo that intracerebroventricular administration of Ghrelin increases bladder capacity dose dependently.

It is likely that ghrelin acts through the second messenger cAMP. Activation of this signal pathway causes relaxation of smooth muscles by decreasing the activity of miosinkinase and stimulating Ca^{2+}-efflux. This effect of ghrelin could be explained with interactions between the two types of transduction pathways, which have opposite effects (Rasmussen & Rasmussen, 1990; Churchill, 1985).

3.2. Gastro-intestinal tract

Angiotensin II

Angiotensin II has potent contractile effect on smooth muscles in the gastro-intestinal tract (GIT). The question for the exact effects of Ang II on GIT remains still opened. Local RAS or parts of it had been found in rat rectum (De Godoy et al., 2006), rat small intestine, and in the guinea pig gall bladder (Leung et al., 1993). The role of Ang II had been confirmed in the development of diseases such as the gastro-esophageal reflux (Fändriks, 2010), incontinence of internal anal sphincter (De Godoy et al., 2006; Rattan et al., 2003), and Crohn's disease (Fändriks, 2010; Wang et al, 1993) as well as other inflammatory and motility disorders of the GIT (Fändriks, 2010).

Most of the effects of Ang II concerning the smooth muscle contractile activity of GIT are associated with AT1 receptors (Fändriks, 2010; Fan et al., 2002; Hawcock & Barnes, 1993; Rattan et al., 2003). AT2 receptors are also described in GIT (Fändriks, 2010; Fan et al., 2002; De Godoy et al., 2006; Hawcock & Barnes, 1993; Ewert et al., 2003; Leung et al., 1993; De Godoy et al., 2002). Although different signaling pathways have been assumed, for example activation of various phosphatases, cGMP -NO system etc. (Ewert et al., 2003; Dinh et al., 2001), their actual signal transduction is not quite elucidated. AT2 receptors are associated with the exchange of water and salts, sodium hydrogen carbonate secretion in the duodenum (Fändriks, 2010) and the secretion of nitric oxide in pig's jejunum (Ewert et al., 2003). The significance of AT2 receptors for GIT motility has not been established yet. It is supposed that they have the opposite effect of AT1 receptors (Gallinat et al., 2000), but as a factor for the smooth muscle relaxation they had been proved only for the internal anal sphincter (De Godoy et al., 2006; De Godoy & Rattan, 2005).

There is not enough information in the literature, regarding to the comparative characteristics of Ang II - induced responses from the various segments of GIT. Dose - dependent curves, which are commonly used as a method for studying the provoked smooth muscle contractions (Fändriks, 2010; Fan et al., 2002; Hawcock & Barnes, 1993; Leung et al., 1993; Park et al., 1973), could give information about the effective doses and maximal responses, but not a data for other important characteristics of the smooth muscle contractions. The different phases of the contraction in the various segments of the GIT, were not clarified and analyzed by application of a time-parameter analysis, as it was made in the study of the skeletal muscle contraction (Raikova & Aladjov, 2004). For comparison and detailed analysis of Ang II contractile effects of Ang II on the different segments of longitudinal strips from rat GIT we are using again time-parameters.

The amplitudes and integral muscle force of different segments from GIT in our experimental study showed marked correlation ($r=0.88$, $p<0.005$). The duodenal muscle strip demonstrated the lowest amplitude and smallest integral force of contraction - 0.55±0.13 g, 41.43±15.52 gs. The amplitudes of the registered angiotensin II-induced contraction from stomach (1.14±0.13 g), jejunum (1.11±0.14 g) and ileum (1.09±0.16 g) are similar and there are not statistically significant differences between them. But stomach integral force (178.09±19.63 gs) is significantly greater than that of duodenum and other intestines and is equally powerful as that of the colon. Under influence of Angiotensin II, rectum developed highest amplitude of contraction 4.74±0.65 g and most powerful integral force - 328.43±75.23 gs.

The analysis of time parameters of Ang II-mediated contractions indicated that the gastric response to Ang II required more time to develop: the time to reach T_{hc} and T_c parameters was 29.09± 2.53 s and 78.18 ± 5.87 s respectively. This tendency for a slower progress of the reaction was maintained during the whole contraction of the stomach and its T_{chr} was 224.90 ± 18.45s. All of the registered intestinal contractions showed similar values for T_{hc} and T_c parameters. For the remaining two time - parameters - T_{hr} and T_{chr}, the results from the intestinal contractions were analogous, with exception of the ileac contraction, which T_{hr} (106.33±9.89 s) and T_{chr} (141.08±9.48 s) were significantly prolonged. After normalization of time-parameter, it was shown that jejunum and colon have similar pattern of contractions and relaxation (Figure 3). The relaxation takes one half of the process and the first and the second part of the contraction are with almost identical proportion, The other parts of GIT - stomach, duodenum and rectum have almost similar pattern of contractions and relaxations. Only ilium differs from these two groups. The relative part of its relaxation was 0.75 from whole duration of process. Application of the time parameters clearly shows the presence of bilateral symmetry in the responses of the gastrointestinal tract.

The amplitude comparison of the Ang II-induced contractions divides the isolated smooth muscle preparations into two groups. The stomach and the small intestines form one group, and the large intestines form another. It is obvious that the large intestines are more sensitive to Ang II and react with more powerful contractions. There is a gradual increase in

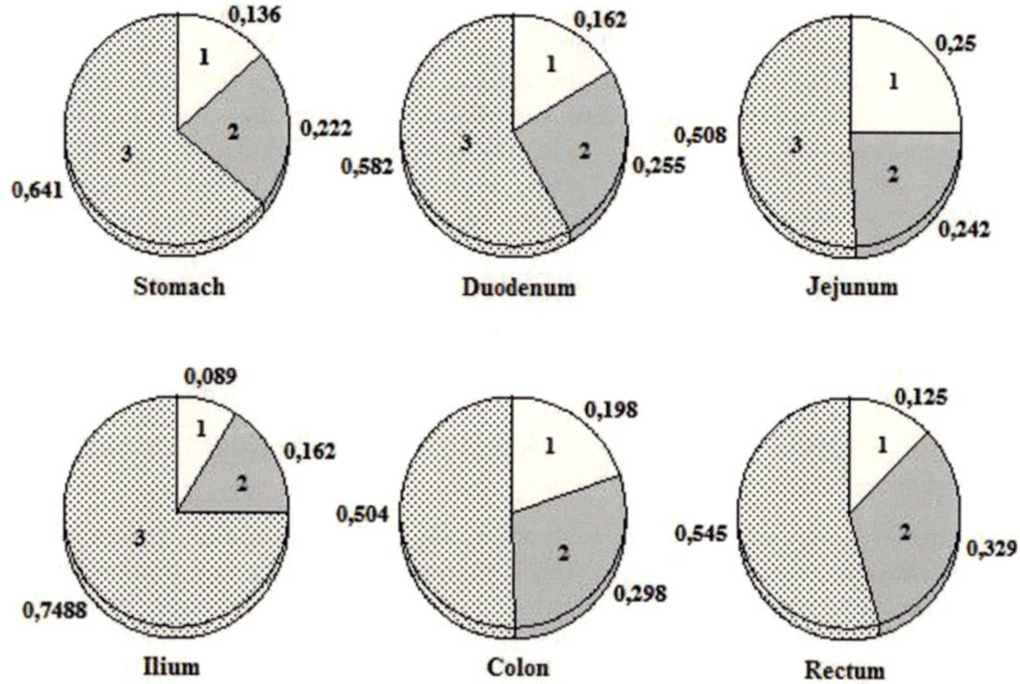

Figure 3. Normalized time-parameters of contractile activity of different GIT segments, induced by Angiotensin II. 1-T_{hcn}, 2-$T_{(c-hc)n}$ and T_{hrn}.

the muscle response to Ang II along the rat intestine, which confirms previous studies of Ang II - provoked intestinal contractions (Ewert et al., 2006). In the literature there are evidences about the uneven distribution of the Ang II receptors in most tissues of the adult organism (Steckelings et al., 2010). Regarding GIT there has been described an unequal density of AT1 receptors (Fändriks, 2010), which could explain the obtained results. From the other side, the duodenal contraction has the smallest amplitude, which strongly differentiates the reaction of the duodenum from the other GIT segments. This could be due to low density of duodenal Ang II receptors and with a local production of NO by the duodenal mucosa (Aihara et al., 2005).

There had been established several transduction pathways of Ang II- induced SMC (Dinh et al., 2001; Romero et al., 1998). The modulating effect of Ang II on different ion currents also had been reported (Chorvatova et al., 1996; Romero et al., 1998). According to T_{hc} and T_c parameters, there is a marked difference between the stomach from the one side, and the intestines from the other. All of the studied intestinal segments showed similar speed of contraction, while the duration of the stomach reaction was far longer. That data suggest a possible transduction pathway for SMC of the stomach, different than in the others GIT segments.

Some authors consider possible competitive interactions between AT1 and AT2 receptors in smooth musculature of the intestine, which supports some previous statements that the magnitude of the response to Ang II depends on the expression of both receptors (Ewert et al., 2006). It had been demonstrated that only AT1 receptors are relevant for the maximum response in ANG-induced contractions (Hawcock & Barnes, 1993; Fändriks, 2010; Fan et al., 2002; Rattan et al., 2003; Ewert et al., 2006; Fändriks, 2010). Despite the existing assumptions that stimulation of AT2 receptors may have the opposite effect than that of AT1 (Gallinat et al., 2000), the role of AT2 receptors for the relaxation phase of the SMC in GIT is not examined. The importance of AT2 receptors for the relaxation of the rectum has been described only (De Godoy et al., 2006; De Godoy & Rattan, 2005). Regarding the time parameters for relaxation, the stomach again showed the slowest response. In this case the ileum indicated significantly prolonged reaction compared to the other intestinal segments. The reason for that difference may be the complete absence or the low density of AT 2 receptors in the ileum (Fändriks, 2010).

In conclusions the observed differences in the Ang II - induced gastro-intestinal contractions may be due to:

- Variation in the Ang II receptor subtypes distribution. Regarding GIT there has been described an unequal density of Ang II receptors. This uneven distribution of the receptors could explain the differences in the amplitude and duration of T_{hc} of SMC.
- Counteraction between Ang II receptor subtypes. Competing actions between Ang II receptors have been discussed in the smooth musculature of rat small intestine. The relative receptor expression is a determinant of the magnitude of response to Ang II. This might be of importance for the duration of muscle contraction after reaching the maximal response - expressed by T_{hr}.
- Activation of various transduction pathways. There is data that Ang II can modulate ionic conductance in distinct tissues. The different duration of the interval between T_{hc} and T_c, as well as T_{hr} may be due to the involvement of some membrane ion channels.
- Presence of local rennin - angiotensin system and formation of numerous of active angiotensin derivates. It is proven that most tissues are the source, target and degradation site of Ang II. Furthermore, local rennin - angiotensin system or parts of it had been found in rat rectum and rat small intestine. This is another possibility which could explain the obtained data about the phase of relaxation and force of SMC.
- The use of time - parameters significantly contributes to the analysis of the contraction process and permits a good comparison of the Ang II – induced responses. Presentation of the time parameters as part of the total contraction normalization) gives an idea for the development of the process in the different time intervals.
- The obtained results provide a direction for further research work on Ang II-mediated contractions of GIT and for clarifying the exact role of the AT1 and AT2 receptors in the different phases of SMC.

Ang II – provoked rectal response. Comparison with the urinary bladder response

The application of Ang II on the rectal preparation caused a development of expressed tonic contraction, which amplitude and integral muscle force were significantly greater than those of the bladder. The higher amplitude is achieved at the expense of the second half of the contraction. The higher values of the absolute and normalized time – parameters for this interval are the evidence. The difference in the total muscle mass of the preparations significantly contributes for these distinctive force parameters. It is worth noted, that the time-parameters (absolute and normalized) of Ang II – mediated bladder and rectal SMC, with the exception of $T_{(c\text{-}hc)}$ parameter, do not indicate significant differences (Figure 4). This proves the suggestion that in the urinary bladder and rectum the Ang II - mediated contractions are developed by similar mechanisms. Moreover, this assumption is an indirect evidence for an approximately equal density of Ang II receptors in these two organs. The uniformity of response to Ang II is supported by the fact that it the rectum a local renin-angiotensin system has also been established (De Godoy & Rattan, 2006). It could be considered again that the locally generated metabolites of Ang II contribute for this pattern of the contraction process.

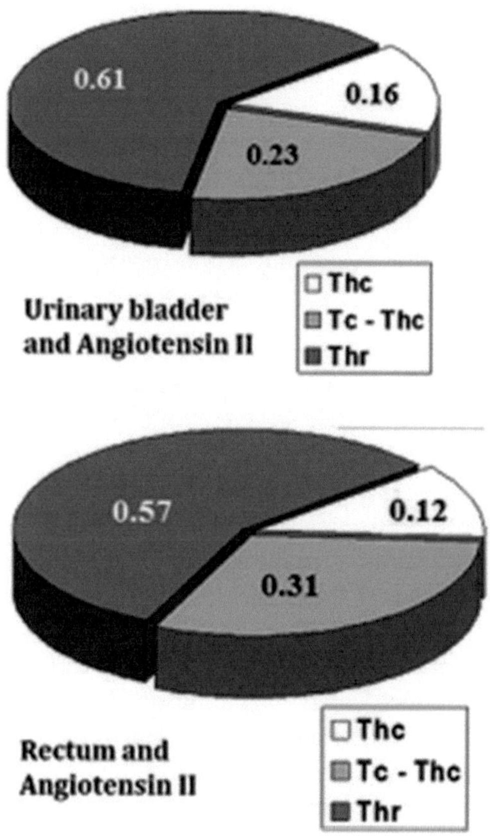

Figure 4. Normalized time-parameters of urinary bladder and rectum Ang II – induced contractions. All of the normalized time-intervals were calculated as a relative part from Tchr.

Does AVP have an importance for the motility of the gastro-intestinal tract?

Dose-dependent effects of AVP on gastro-intestinal tract from different species were observed, but regarding the rectal musculature the information is insufficient and controversial (Ohlsson et al., 2006). AVP has been shown to increase the gastric and duodenal motility in humans and rabbits (Ohlsson et al., 2006; Li et al., 2007), as well as colonic peristalsis, but the expression of the AVP receptors in intestine has not been examined yet (Ohlsson et al., 2006). Some authors have demonstrated that AVP increase the gastro-intestinal motility via the oxytocin OT1 receptors, but the experiment is only for stomach and duodenum from rabbits (Li et al., 2007).

In our study, the application of AVP does not significantly alter the characteristics of the spontaneous phasic contractile activity of gastro-intestinal segments except this of stomach. This could be explained with the absence of AVP receptors type V1, which are present in the urinary bladder. In rectal musculature V2 receptors could be presented – in such a case, the rectum as a terminal department of gastro-intestinal tract shows analogy with the distal and the collecting tubules of the kidneys. This is still an assumption that remains to be investigated.

Gallbladder

The mechanical activity of the gallbladder of conscious dogs consisted of spontaneous rhythmic contractions with a frequency of 2 to 5 cpm. Fluctuations of the tone were also observed. Bolus injection of cholecystokinin octapeptide i.v. produced a dose-dependent increase in gallbladder pressure (Figure 5A). Atropine decreased gallbladder pressure and reduced or even abolished the cholecystokinin action (Figure 5B). Hexamethonium led to gallbladder relaxation and also greatly reduced the gallbladder response to cholecystokinin octapeptide (Figure 5C).

The mechanisms through which atropine or hexamethonium inhibit cholecystokinin-produced gallbladder contractions under in vivo conditions are not understood. One possible explanation might be that the excitatory effect of cholecystokinin on the gallbladder is mediated by acetylcholine release from cholinergic neurons at pre- and post- ganglionic level. Another possibility is that atropine and/or hexamethonium are able to block the release of endogenous cholecystokinin from the endocrine cells or neurons. This suggestion is supported by the fact that vagotomy abolish gallbladder response to cholecystokinin after acidification (Fried et al., 1983), infusion of fat into the duodenum (Magee et al., 1984) or after drinking water (Sundler et al., 1977). The release of CCK in the circulation in response to fat or other meals is also reduced after vagotomy or atropine. It is also possible that atropine or hexamethonium blockade of cholinergic input to the gallbladder may unmask the release of neuronal inhibitory influence which could then compete with the release of CCK. Such inhibitory agents could be somatostatin and vasoactive intestinal peptide (Lenz et al., 1993; Milenov et al., 1995).

Uterus

It has been reported that in the uteri of a number of species, local production of Ang II and the enzymes for its synthesis are present. Besides the proven contractile effect of Ang II on the uterine arteries, research in this area showed that myometrium is also sensitive to the effect of this octapeptide (Keskil et al., 1999).

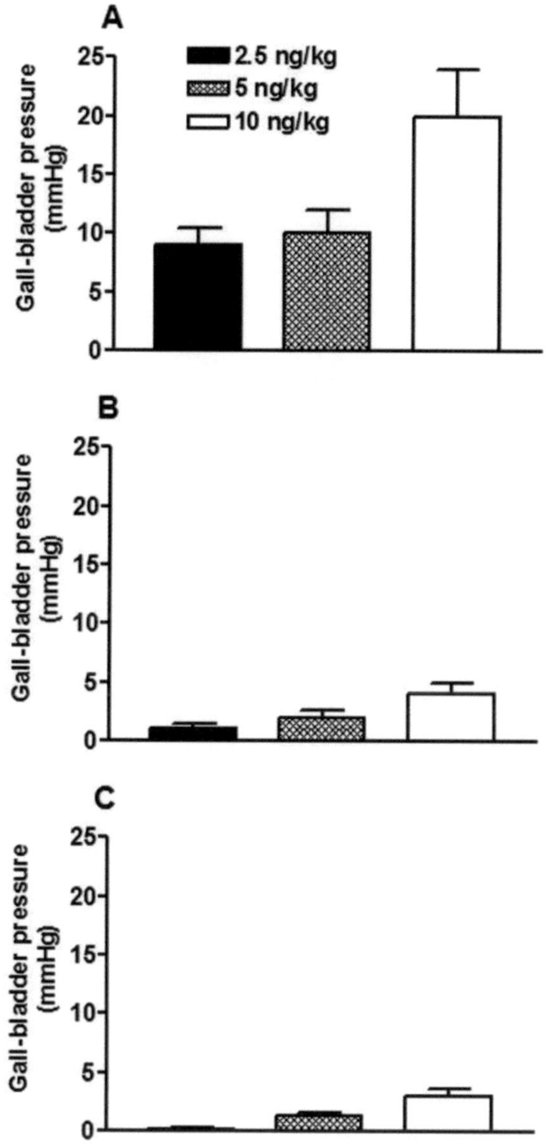

Figure 5. CCK-8 (2.5; 5 and 10 ng/kg i.v.)-induced gallbladder pressure before (A) and after atropine (B) (20 μg/kg i.v.) or hexamethonium (C) (1 mg/kg i.v.). Means ± S.E.M. of 12 experiments in 6 conscious dogs are presented, $P < 0.01$.

There is substantial evidence for the involvement of AVP in conditions of uterine hyperactivity. Even more, it has been shown that the human myometrium is more sensitive to AVP than to oxytocin (Bossmar et al., 2007).

Ang II at concentration of 1 μmol induced tonic contraction with maximum amplitude of 6.00 ± 0.22 g and an integral force of muscle contraction of 1150.00 ± 614.70 gs. AVP applied in the same concentration as Ang II induced tonic contractions with amplitude of 6.61 ± 0.39 g (n = 8) and an integral force of muscle contraction of 7245.00 ±901.00 gs. The duration of the AVP-induced responses was several times greater than those of Ang II and the recording of AVP-mediated contractions was stopped on the 30th minute without achievement of T_{chr} parameter.

Our experiment confirmed the contractile effect of these two peptides on the myometrium, which is in accordance with the results of other authors working on the same issues (Anouar et al., 1996; Chan et al., 1996; Keskil et al., 1999).

The contractions induced by both peptides have similar amplitudes, but they are with different duration and characteristics. The registered AVP - provoked uterine responses were found to have a sustained oscillating character Figure 6). When analyzed by mathematical modeling such contractions were recognized as underdamped process - the system tries to establish a stable level different from the baseline (Yankov, 2009). The differences in the developed contractions may be due to split of the classical or inclusion of additional transduction pathway for each of the studied peptides. Both of them have several main groups of receptors. The receptors for Ang II are AT1 and AT2 (De Gasparo et al., 2000), while the receptors for AVP are V1a, V1b and V2 (Petersen, 2006).

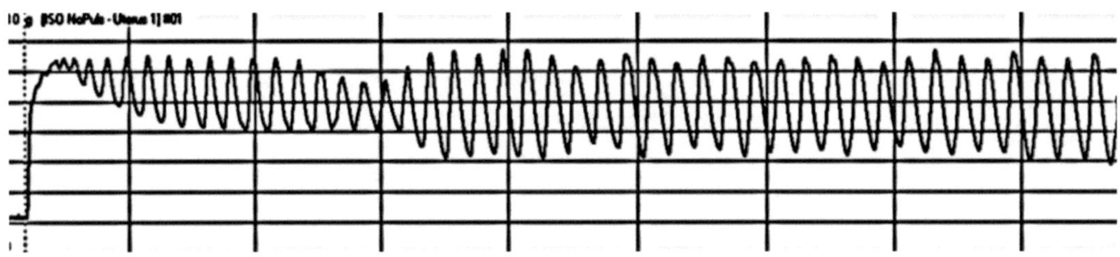

Figure 6. Original record of vasopressin-induced uterine contraction.

To establish the importance of these receptors for the uterine muscle contraction will be the subject of our next experiments. However, several interesting facts immerge:

First – the constrictor effect of Ang II is associated with AT1 receptors, but the uterus is one of the few organs with a. uterina inferior where AT2 receptors are predominant (Keskil et al., 1999). AT2 receptors are mainly regarded to oppose the effects of AT1 and cause dilation, blood pressure reduction, nitric oxide production (Hannan et al., 2003). Perhaps the significantly shorter phase of contraction and relaxation was due to their activation under the influence of Ang II in the uterus. Second – the constrictor effect of AVP is realized by V1a receptors which are found in uterine arteries. With regard to the contractile response of the myometrium, however, there are statements that the resulting contraction from the AVP influence is due to activation of other receptors, different from the mentioned above (Anouar et al., 1996). Some authors go even further and argue that AVP accomplish its effect on uterine musculature by OT receptors, which have big similarity with V1 receptors (Chan et al., 1996).

Considering that both peptides are released from supraoptic nuclei in the hypothalamus and that they have a powerful contractile effect on the smooth muscle, it is appropriate to search a closer connection between them in preparing the uterus for pregnancy and labor. Probably these two peptides act synchronously which potentiate their own effects (Douglas et al.,2001).

Studies on rats show that AVP is more potent uterotonic agent than OT in non pregnant condition (Bossmar et al., 2007) and during parturition OT predominantly promotes uterine contractions, while AVP is more important for vasoconstriction, thus reducing the bleeding after delivery (Chan et al., 1996; Douglas et al.,2001).

The study of Ang II – and AVP – mediated uterine contractions contributes considerably for the revealing of the mechanisms that generate and modulate uterine activity. This could be beneficial for a better understanding and control of myometrial dysfunction.

Author details

Anna Tolekova, Petya Hadzhibozheva, Tsvetelin Georgiev, Stanislava Mihailova and Galina Ilieva
Department of Physiology, Pathophysiology and Pharmacology, Medical Faculty, Trakia University, Stara Zagora, Bulgaria

Maya Gulubova
Department of General and Clinical Pathology, Medical Faculty, Trakia University, Stara Zagora, Bulgaria

Eleonora Leventieva-Necheva, Kiril Milenov and Reni Kalfin
Institute of Neurobiology, Bulgarian Academy of Sciences, Sofia, Bulgaria

Acknowledgement

This work was supported by Grant DDVU-02-24/2010 from the National Science Fund, Sofia, Bulgaria and Grant MF - 1/2010 from Medical Faculty, Trakia University.

5. References

Aguilera G (1994) Regulation of pituitary ACTH secretion during chronic stress. Front Neuroendocrinol.,15:321-50.

Aihara E, Kagawa S, Hayashi M & Takeuchi K (2005) ACE inhibitor and AT1 antagonist stimulate duodenal HCO3- secretion mediated by a common pathway - involvement of PG, NO and bradykinin. J Physiol Pharmacol, 563: 391-406.

Allen AM, MacGregor DP, McKinley MJ, Mendelsohn FA (1999) Angiotensin II receptors in the human brain. Regul Pept, 79:1–7.

Andersson KE & Arner A (2004) Urinary bladder contraction and relaxation: physiology and pathophysiology. Physiol Rev, 84: 935-986.

Andersson KE, Hedlund H & Stahl M (1992) Contractions induced by angiotensin I, angiotensin II and bradykinin in isolated smooth muscle from the human detrusor. Acta Physiol Scand, 145(3): 253-259.

Andersson KE, Husted S, Mattiasson A & Maller-Madsen B (1982) Atropine resistance of trasmurally stimulated isolated human bladder muscle. Urol Res, 15: 355-358.

Anouar A, Clerget M, Durroux T, Barberis C, Germain G (1996) Comparison of vasopressin and oxytocin receptors in the rat uterus and vascular tissue. Eur J Pharmacol, 308(1): 87-96

Armstead W (2001) Vasopressin-induced protein kinase C-dependent superoxide generation conributes to ATP- sensitive potassium channel but not calcium- sensitive potassium channel function impairment after brain injury. Stroke, 326: 1408-1414.

Barassin S, Kalsbeek A, Saboureau M, Bothorel B, Vivien-Roels B, Malan A, Buijs RM, Pevet P (2000) Potentiation effect of vasopressin on melatonin secretion as determined by trans-pineal microdialysis in the Rat. J Neuroendocrinol., 121:61-8.

Becke C, Thiebot MH, Touitou Y, Hamon M, Cesselin F, Benoliel JJ (2001). Enhanced cortical extracellular levels of cholecystokinin-like material in a model of anticipation of social defeat in the rat. J Neurosci 21: 262–269.

Berridge M (2008) Smooth muscle cell calcium activation mechanisms. J Physiol, 586: 5047-5061.

Bosch OJ, Neumann ID (2008) Brain vasopressin is an important regulator of maternal behavior independent of dams' trait anxiety. Proc Natl Acad Sci U S A,105(44):17139-44.

Bossmar T, Osman N, Zilahi E, Haj M, Nowotny N, Conlon J (2007) Expression of the oxytocin gene, but not the vasopressin gene, in the rat uterus during pregnancy: influence of oestradiol and progesterone. J Endocrinol, 193: 121-126.

Briley EM, Lolait SJ, Axelrod J, Felder CC (1994) The cloned vasopressin V1a receptor stimulates phospholipase A2, phospholipase C, and phospholipase D through activation of receptor-operated calcium channels. Neuropeptides, 27: 63-74.

Broglio F, Arvat E, Benso A, Papotti M, Miccioli G, Deghenghi R, Ghigo E. (2002) Ghrelin: Endocrine and Non-endocrine Actions J Ped Endocrinol & Metab, 15: 1219-1227.

Broglio F, Gottero C, Arvat E, Ghigo E (2003) Endocrine and Non-endocrine of Ghrelin. Horm Res, 59: 109–117.

Burnstock G (1990) In: Neurobiology of Incontinence: Innervation of bladder and bowel. Ciba Foundation Symposium 151: 2-26, Chichester, Wiley.

Callahan SM, Creed KE (1986) Non-cholinergic neurotransmission and the effects of peptides on the urinary bladder of guinea-pigs and rabbits. J Physiol, 374: 103-115.

Cantor P (1986) Evaluation of a radioimmunoassay for cholecystokinin in human plasma. Scand J Clin Lab Invest, 46: 213-221.

Chan W, Wo N, Manning M (1996) The role of oxytocin receptors and vasopressin V1a receptors in uterine contractions in rats: implications for tocolytic therapy with oxytocin antagonists. Am J Obstet Gynecol, 175(5): 1331-1335.

Chen TF, Doyle PT & Ferguson DR (1994) Inhibition in the human urinary bladder by gamma-amino-butyric acid. Br J Urol, 73: 250-255.

Chiu AT, Smith RD, Timmermans PB (1994) Defining Angiotensin Receptor Subtypes. In: J.M. Saavedra & P.B. Timmermans Eds.), Angiotensin Receptors 1st edition, 49-65). New York: Springer-Verlag.

Chorvatova A, Gallo-Payet N, Casanova C, Payet MD (1996) Modulation of membrane potential and ionic currents by the AT1 and AT2 receptors of angiotensin II. Cell Signal, 88: 525-32.

Churchill PC (1985) Second messengers in renin secretion. Am J Physiol Renal Physiol, 249: F175-84.

Cohen SL, Knight M, Tamminga CA, Chase TN (1982). Cholecystokinin-octapeptide effects on conditioned-avoidance behavior, stereotypy and catalepsy. Eur J Pharmacol 83: 213-222.

Compaan JC, Buijs RM, Pool CW, De Ruiter AJ, Koolhaas JM (1993) Differential lateral septal vasopressin innervation in aggressive and nonaggressive male mice. Brain Res Bull., 301(2):1-6.

Crankshaw DJ (1989) (Arg^{8}) vasopressin-induces contractions of rabbit urinary bladder smooth muscle. Eur J Pharmacol, 173(2-3): 183-8.

Crawley JN, Corwin RL (1994). Biological actions of cholecystokinin. Peptides, 154: 731-755.

Crawley JN (1992). Subtype-selective cholecystokinin receptor antagonists block cholecystokinin modulation of dopamine-mediated behaviors in the rat mesolimbic pathway. J Neurosci, 12: 3380-3391.

Crespi F, Corsi M, Reggiani A, Ratti E, Gaviraghi G (2000). Involvement of cholecystokinin within craving for cocaine: role of cholecystokinin receptor ligands. Exp Opin Invest Drugs, 9: 2249–2258.

Crowe R, Burnstock G (1989). A histochemical and immuno-histochemical study of the autonomic innervation of the lower urinary tract of the female pig. Is the pig a good model for the human bladder and urethra? J Urol, 141: 414-422.

Date Y, Nakazato M, Hashiguchi S, Dezaki K, Mondal MS, Hosoda H, Kojima M, Kangawa K, Arima T, Matsuo H, Yada T & Matsukura S (2002) Ghrelin is present in pancreatic alpha-cells of humans and rats and stimulates insulin secretion. Diabetes, 51(1): 124–129.

Davenport AP, Bonner TI, Foord SM, Harmar AJ, Neubig RR, Pin JP, Spedding M, Kojima M, Kangawa K (2005) International Union of Pharmacology. LVI. Ghrelin Receptor Nomenclature, Distribution and Function. Pharmacol Rev, 57: 541-546.

De Gasparo M, Catt K, Inagami T, Wright J, Unger T (2000) International union of pharmacology. XXIII. The angiotensin II receptors. Pharmacol Rev, 52(3): 415-72.

De Godoy MA, Rattan S (2005) Autocrine regulation of internal anal sphincter tone by renin-angiotensin system: comparison with phasic smooth muscle. Am J Physiol Gastrointest Liver Physiol, 289(6): G1164-75, b.

De Godoy MA, Rattan S (2006) Angiotensin-converting enzyme and angiotensin II receptor subtype 1 inhibitors restitute hypertensive internal anal sphincter in the spontaneously hypertensive rats. J Pharmacol Exp Ther, 318(2): 725-34, a.

De Godoy MA, Dunn S, Rattan S (2004) Evidence for the role of angiotensin II biosynthesis in the rat internal anal sphincter tone. Gastroenterology, 127(1): 127-38.

De Godoy MA, Rattan S (2006) Translocation of AT1- and AT2-receptors by higher concentrations of angiotensin II in the smooth muscle cells of rat internal anal sphincter. J Pharmacol Exp Ther, 319(3): 1088-95.

De Groat WC, Booth AM (1984) In: Peripheral Neuropathy: Autonomic systems to the urinary bladder and sexual organs. P.J. Dyck, P.K. Thomas, E.H. Lambert & R. Bunge (eds), Philadelphia, W.B. Saunders, 285-299.

De Groat WC, Booth AM (1993) In: Nervous control of the urogenital system: Synaptic transmission in pelvic ganglia. Maggi CA (ed), Harwood Academic Publ, Chur, 291-347.

De Groat WC, Kawatani M (1985) Neural control of the urinary bladder: Possible relationship between peptidergic inhibitory mechanisms and detrusor instability. Neurourol Urodyn, 4: 285-300.

Degen L., Matzinger, D., Drewe, J., Beglinger, C (2001). The effect of cholecystokinin in controlling appetite and food intake in humans. Peptides, 22: 1265–1269.

Dehpour AR, Kivaj GRT, Delfan A, Shahrokhi M (1997) The effects of lithium, indomethacine and neomycin on vassopresin-inducted contractions in rat urinary bladder. Gen Pharmacol, 28(5): 777-780.

Dinh DT, Frauman AG, Johnston CI, Fabiani ME (2001) Angiotensin receptors: distribution, signalling and function. Clin Sci (Lond), 100(5): 481-92.

Dixon JS, Jen PY, Gosling JA (1997) A double-label immunohisto-chemical study of intramural ganglia from the human male urinary bladder neck. J Anat, 190: 125-134.

Dornan WA, Malsbury CW (1989) Peptidergic control of male sexual behavior: the effects of intracerebral injections of substance P and cholecystokinin. Physiol Behav, 46: 547–56.

Douglas A, Scullion S, Antonijevic I, Brown D, Russell J, Leng G (2001) Uterine contractile activity stimulates supraoptic neurons in term pregnant rats via a noradrenergic pathway. Endocrinology, 142(2): 633-44.

Downie JW (1981) The autonomic pharmacology of the urinary bladder and urethra: a neglected area. Trends Pharmacol Sci, 2: 163-165.

Dufresne M, Seva C, Fourmy D (2006) Cholecystokinin and gastrin receptors. Physiol Rev, 86(3): 805–847.

Eva C, Oberto A, Mele P, Serra M, Biggio G (2006) Role of brain neuroactive steroids in the functional interplay between the GABAA and the NPY-Y1 receptor mediated signals in the Amygdala. Pharmacology Biochemistry and Behavior, 84 (4): 568–580.

Ewert S, Laesser M, Johansson B, Holm M, Aneman A, Fandriks L (2003) The angiotensin II receptor type 2 agonist CGP 42112A stimulates NO production in the porcine jejunal mucosa. BMC Pharmacol, 3:2.

Ewert S, Spak E, Olbers T, Johnsson E, Edebo A, Fändriks L (2006) Angiotensin II induced contraction of rat and human small intestinal wall musculature in vitro. Acta Physiol (Oxf), 188(1): 33-40.

Fan YP, Puri RN, Rattan S (2002) Animal model for angiotensin II effects in the internal anal sphincter smooth muscle: mechanism of action. Am J Physiol Gastrointest Liver Physiol, 282(3): G461-9.

Fändriks L (2010) The angiotensin II type 2 receptor and the gastrointestinal tract. J Renin Angiotensin Aldosterone Syst., 11(1): 43-8.

Feher E, Vajda J (1981) Sympathetic innervation of the urinary bladder. Acta Morphol Acad Sci Hung, 29: 27-35.

Ferens D, Yin L, Ohashi-Doi K, Habgood M, Bron R, Brock J, Gale J, Furness J (2010) Evidence for functional ghrelin receptors on parasympathetic preganglionic neurons of micturition control pathways in the rat. Clin Exp Pharmacol Physiol, 37 (9): 926–932.

Fitts DA, Starbuck EM and Ruhf A (2000) Circumventricular organs and Ang II-induced salt appetite: blood pressure and connectivity. Am J Physiol, Reg Integ Comp Physiol, 279: R2277-R2286.

Frank E, Landgraf R (2008) The vasopressin system--from antidiuresis to psychopathology. Eur J Pharmacol.,583(2-3):226-42.

Fried GM, Ogden WD, Greely GG (1983) Correlation of release and action of cholecystokinin in dogs before and after vagotomy. Surgery, 93(6): 786-792.

Fujino K, Inui A, Asakawa A, Kihara N, Fujimura M, Fujimiya M (2003) Ghrelin induced fasted motor activity of the gastrointestinal tract in conscious fed rats. J Physiol, 550(1): 227-240.

Gabella G, Uvelius B (1990) Urinary bladder of rat: fine structure of normal and hypertrophic musculature. Cell Tissue Res, 262: 67-79.

Gagnon DJ, Sirois P (1972) The rat isolated colon as a specific assay organ for angiotensin. Br J Pharmacol, 46(1): 89-93.

Gallinat S, Busche S, Raizada MK, Sumners C (2000) The angiotensin II type 2 receptor: an enigma with multiple variations. Am J Physiol Endocrinol Metab, 278(3): E357-74.

García M, López M, Alvarez C, Casanueva F, Tena-Sempere M, Diéguez C (2007) Role of ghrelin in reproduction. Reproduction, 133(3): 531–540.

Ge J, Barnes NM (1996) Alterations in angiotensin AT1 and AT2 receptor subtype levels in brain regions from patients with neurodegenerative disorders. Eur J Pharmacol, 297: 299-306.

Georgiev V, Yonkov D (1985) Participation of angiotensin II in learning and memory: I. Interaction of angiotensin II with saralasin.Meth Find Exp Clin Pharmacol, 7: 415-418.

Ghigo E, Broglio F Arvat E, Maccario M, Paoti M, Muccioli G (2005) Ghrelin: more than a natural GH secretagoue and/or an orexigenic factor. Clin Endocrinol, 62: 1-17.

Goncharuk VD, Buijs RM, Jhamandas JH, Swaab DF (2011) Vasopressin (VP) and neuropeptide FF (NPFF) systems in the normal and hypertensive human brainstem. J Comp Neurol, 519(1):93-124.

Goodson JL, Bass AH (2001) Social behavior functions and related anatomical characteristics of vasotocin/vasopressin systems in vertebrates. Brain Res Brain Res Rev, 35(3):246-65.

Gulubova MV, Hadjipetkov P, Sivrev D, Ilieva G (2012) Endocrine cells in the human common bile duct in patients with obstructive jaundice. Hepatogastroenterology, 59(113): 26-30

Hadzhibozheva P, Iliev R, Tolekova A, Ilieva G, Trifonova K, Sandeva R, Tsokeva Z, Kalfin R (2009) Effects of some neuropeptide on detrusor strips from rat urinary bladder. Bulg J Vet Med, 12: 67-72.

Hannan R, Davis E, Widdop R (2003) Functional role of angiotensin II AT2 receptor in modulation of AT1 receptor-mediated contraction in rat uterine artery: involvement of bradykinin and nitric oxide. Br J Pharmacol, 140(5): 987-95.

Harper AA, Raper HS (1943) Pancreozymin, a stimulant of the secretion of pancreatic enzymes in extracts of the small intestine. J Physiol, 102: 115-125.

Hashimoto H, Ueta Y (2011) Central effects of ghrelin, a unique peptide, on appetite and fluid/water drinking behavior. Curr Protein Pept Sci., 12(4) : 280-7.

Hawcock AB, Barnes JC (1993) Pharmacological characterization of the contractile responses to angiotensin analogues in guinea-pig isolated longitudinal muscle of small intestine. Br J Pharmacol, 108(4): 1150-5.

Helm G, Owman C, Rosengren E, Sjoberg NO (1982) Regional and cyclic variations in catecholamine concentration of the human fallopian tube. Biol Reprod, 26: 553-558.

Hermes ML, Ruijter JM, Klop A, Buijs RM, Renaud LP (2000)Vasopressin increases GABAergic inhibition of rat hypothalamic paraventricular nucleus neurons in vitro. J Neurophysiol, 83(2):705-11.

Hokfelt T, Rehfeld JF, Skirboll L, Ivemark B, Goldstein M, Markey K (1980) Evidence for coexistence of dopamine and CCK in meso-limbic neurones. Nature, 285: 476–478.

Holmes CL, Patel BM, Russell JA, Walley KR (2001) The physiology of vasopresin relevant to the management of septic shock. Chest,120: 989-1002.

Ilieva G, Tolekova A, Sandeva R, Trifonova K, Tsokeva Zh, Ganeva M (2008) Influence of ghrelin on Angiotensin II mediated contraction of smooth muscle strips from urinary bladder. Trakia J Sci, 6(2): 77-81,a.

Ilieva G, Tolekova A, Sandeva R, Trifonova K, Tsokeva Zh, Ganeva M, Mihova Z, Tolev A, Zezovski S (2008) Role of transmembrane calcium current in angiotensin II – mediated contraction of detrusor organ strips from rat urinary bladder. Bulg J Vet Med, 11(2): 89-94.

Inui A, Asakawa A, Bowers CY, Mantovani G, Laviano A, Meguid M, Fujimiya M (2004) Ghrelin, aetite, and gastric motility: the emerging role of the stomach as an endocrine organ. The FASEB Journal,18: 439-456.

Ivy AC, Oldberg E (1928) A hormone mechanism of gall bladder contraction and evacuation. Am J Physiol, 86: 599-613.

Janig W, McLachlan EM (1987) Organization of lumbar spinal outflow to distal colon and pelvic organs. Physiol Rev, 67: 1332-1404.

Josselyn SA, Vaccarino FJ (1996) Acquisition of conditioned reward blocked by intra-accumbens infusion of PD-140548, a CCKA receptor antagonist. Pharmacol Biochem Behav, 55: 439–444.

Kalra S, Dube M, Pu S, Xu B, Horvath TP, Kalra S (1999) Interacting appetite-regulating pathways in the hypothalamic regulation of body weight. Endocrine Reviews, 20 (1): 68–100.

Kalsbeek A, Buijs RM, Engelmann M, Wotjak CT, Landgraf R (1995) In vivo measurement of a diurnal variation in vasopressin release in the rat suprachiasmatic nucleus. Brain Res, 682(1-2):75-82.

Kalsbeek A, Fliers E, Hofman MA, Swaab DF, Buijs RM (2010) Vasopressin and the output of the hypothalamic biological clock. J Neuroendocrinol.,22(5):362-72.

Kam P, Williams S, Yoong F (2004) Vasopressin and terlipressin: pharmacology and its clinical relevance. Anaesthesia, 59: 993-1001.

Kang KS, Yahashi S, Matsuda K (2011) The Effects of Ghrelin on Energy Balance and Psychomotor Activity in a Goldfish International. Journal of Peptides, 1- 9.

Keskil Z, Bayram M, Ercan Z, Türker R (1999) The contribution of nitric oxide and endothelins to angiotensin: II. Evoked responses in the rat isolated uterus smooth muscle. Gen Pharmacol, 33(4): 307-12.

Kim S, Awao H (2011) Molecular and Cellular Mechanisms of Angiotensin II-Mediated Cardiovascular and Renal Diseases. Pharmacological reviews; 52(1): 1-24.

Kim S, Iwao H (2000) Molecular and cellular mechanisms of angiotensin II-mediated cardiovascular and renal diseases. Pharmacol Rev, 52: 11–34.

Kojima M, Kangawa K (2005) Ghrelin: Structure and Function. Physiol Rev., 85:495-522.

Kola B, Hubina E, Tucci S Kirkham TC, Garcia EA, Mitchell SE, Williams LM, Hawley SA, Hardie DG, Grossman AB, Korbonits M (2005) Cannabinoids and ghrelin have both central and peripheral metabolic and cardiac effects via AMP-activated protein kinase. Journal of Biological Chemistry, 280 (26): 25196–25201.

Kovács GL, Bohus B, Versteeg DHG, Kloet ER, Wied D (1979) Effect of oxytocin and vasopressin on memory consolidation: sites of action and catecholaminergic correlates after local microinjection into limbic-midbrain structures. Brain Res, 175: 303-314.

Lasanen LT, Tammela TL, Kallioinen M, Waris T (1992) Effect of acute distension on cholinergic innervation of the rat urinary bladder. Urol Res, 20: 59-62.

Lee H, Wang G, Englander EW, Kojima M, Greeley G (2002) Ghrelin, a new gastrointestinal endocrine peptide that stimulates insulin secretion: enteric distribution, ontogeny, influence of endocrine, and dietary manipulations. Endocrinology, 143(1): 185–190.

Lenkei Z, Palkovits M, Corvol P, Lorens-Cortes C (1997) Expression of angiotensin type-1 (AT1) and type-2 (AT2) receptor mRNA in the adult rat brain: A functional neuroanatomical review. Front Neuroendocrinol, 18: 383-439.

Lenz HJ, Zimmerman FG, Messmer B (1993) Regulation of canine gallbladder motility by brain peptides. Gastroenterology, 104(6): 1678-1685.

Leung E, Ra JM, Walsh LK, Zeitung KD, Eglen RM (1993) Characterization of angiotensin II receptors in smooth muscle preparations of the guinea pig in vitro. J Pharmacol Exp Ther, 267(3): 1521-8.

Li L, Kong X, Liu H, Liu C (2007) Systemic oxytocin and vasopressin excite gastrointestinal motility through oxytocin receptor in rabbits. Neurogastroenterol & Motility, 19(10): 839–844.

Liddle RA (1997) Cholecystokinin cells. Annu Rev Physiol, 59: 221-242.

Lieverse RJ, Masclee AA, Jansen JB, Rovati LC, Lamers CB (1995) Satiety effects of the type A CCK receptor antagonist loxiglumide in lean and obese women. Biol Psychiatry, 37(5): 331-335.

Lim CT, Kola B, Korbonits M, Grossman AB (2010) Ghrelin's role as a major regulator of appetite and its other functions in neuroendocrinology. Prog. Brain Res., 182: 189-205.

Lindberg BF, Nilsson LG, Hedlund H, Stahl M, Andersson KE (1994) Angiotensin I is converted to angiotensin II by a serine protease in human detrusor smooth muscle. Am J Physiol, 266 (6): R1861-1867.

Lu H, Fern R, Luthin D, Linden J, Liu L, Cohen Ch, Barrett P (1996) Angiotensin II stimulates T-type Ca^{2+} channel currents via activation of a G protein, G_i. Am J Physiol, 271 (4): C1340-1349.

Lu S, Guan J, Wang Q, Uehara K, Yamada S, Goto N, Date Y, Nakazato M, Kojima M, Kangawa K, Shioda S (2002) Immunocytochemical observation of ghrelin-containing neurons in the rat arcuate nucleus. Neurosci Lett, 321(3): 157–160.

Luo B, Cheu JW, Siegel A (1998) Cholecystokinin B receptors in the periaqueductal gray potentiate defensive rage behavior elicited from the medial hypothalamus of the cat. Brain Res, 796: 27–37.

Magee DF, Naruse S, Pap A (1984) Vagal control of gallbladder contraction. J Physiol, 355: 65-70.

Mager U, Kolehmainen M, de Mello V, Schwab U, Laaksonen D, Rauramaa R, Gylling H, Atalay M, Pulkkinen L, Uusitupa M (2008) Expression of ghrelin gene in peripheral blood mononuclear cells and plasma ghrelin concentrations in patients with metabolic syndrome. Eur J Endocrinol, 158(4): 499–510.

Maggi AC (1991) The role of peptides in the regulation of the micturition reflex: an update. Gen Pharmacol, 22: 1-24.

Maggi AC (1995) Tachykinins and calcitonin gene-related peptide CGRP) as cotransmitters released from peripheral ending of sensory nerves. Prog Neurobiol, 45: 1-98.

Markowski, VP, Hull EM (1995). Cholecystokinin modulates mesulimbic dopaminergic influences on male rat copulatory behavior. Brain Res, 699: 266–274.

Matsuda K, Kang K, Sakashita A, Yahashi S, Vaudry H (2011) Behavioral effect of neuropeptides related to feeding regulation in fish. Annals of the New York Academy of Sciences, 1220 (1): 117–12.

Matsuta Y, Nagase K, Ishida H, Tanase K, Akino H and Yokoyama O (2011) Peripheral ghrelin administration increases bladder capacity without affecting the bladder contraction pressure or electroencephalogram in rats. Available: http://www.icsoffice.org/Abstracts/Publish/106/000454.pdf

McKinley MJ, Albiston AL, Allen AM, Mathai ML, May CN, McAllen RM, Oldfield BJ, Mendelsohn FAO, Chai SY (2003) The brain renin–angiotensin system: location and physiological roles. The International Journal of Biochemistry & Cell Biology, 35: 901–918.

Milenov K, Rakovska A, Kalfin R (1995) Effects of cholecystokinin on the gallbladder motility: Interaction with somatostatin and vasoactive intestinal peptide. Acta Physiol Pharmacol Bulg 21: 67-76.

Milosević VL, Stevanović DM, Nesić DM, Sosić-Jurjević BT, Ajdzanović VZ, Starcević VP, Severs WB (2010) Central effects of ghrelin on the adrenal cortex: a morphological and hormonal study. Gen Physiol Biophys, 29(2):194-202.

Miyazaki M, Takai S (2006) Tissue angiotensin II generating system by angiotensin-converting enzyme ans chimase. J Pharmacol Sci,100(5): 391-7.

Mladenov M, Hristov K, Duridanova D (2006) Ghrelin Suression of Potassium Currents in Smooth Muscle Cells of Human Mesenteric Artery. Gen Physiol Biophys, 25: 333-338.

Mutt V (1980) Cholecystokinin: Isolation, structure and function. In: Glass GBJ, editor. Gastrointestinal Hormones. New York: Raven Press. 169-203.

Ohlsson B, Björgell O, Ekberg O, Darwiche G (2006) The oxytocin/vasopressin receptor antagonist atosiban delays the gastric emptying of a semisolid meal compared to saline in human. BMC Gastroenterol,16: 6 -11.

Otsuka A, Barnes KL and Ferrario CM (1986) Contribution of area postrema to pressor actions of angiotensin II in dog. Am J Physiol, 251: H538-H546.

Park WK, Regoli D, Rioux F (1973) Characterization of angiotensin receptors in vascular and intestinal smooth muscles. Br J Pharmacol, 48(2): 288-301.

Paul M, Poyan Mehr A, Kreutz R (2006) Physiology of local renin-angiotensin systems. Physiol Rev, 86(3): 747-803.

Petersen M (2006) The effect of vasopressin and related compounds at V1a and V2 receptors in animal models relevant to human disease. Basic Clin Pharmacol Toxicol, 99(2): 96-103

Petkov G, Hener T, Bonev A, Herrera G, Nelson M (2001) Low levels of K_{ATP} channel activation decrease excitability and contractility of urinary bladder. Am J Physiol Regul Integr Comp Physiol, 280 (5): R1427-R1433.

Phull H, Salkini M, Escobar C, Purves T, Comiter CV (2007) The role of angiotensin II in stress urinary incontinence: A rat model. Neurourol Urodyn, 26(1): 81-88.

Pickar J, Hill J, Kaufman MP (1993) Stimulation of vagal afferents inhibits locomotion in mesencephalic cats. Journal of Applied Physiology, 74 (1): 103–110.

Raikova RT, Aladjov HT (2004) Simulation of the motor units control during a fast elbow flexion in the sagittal plane. J Electromyogr Kinesiol, 14(2): 227-38.

Rasmussen H, Rasmussen JE (1990) Calcium as intracellular messenger: From simplicity to Complexity. Curr Top Cell Regul, 31: 1-109.

Rattan S, Puri RN, Fan YP (2003) Involvement of rho and rho-associated kinase in sphincteric smooth muscle contraction by angiotensin II. Exp Biol Med (Maywood), 228(8): 972-81.

Romero F, Silva BA, Nouailhetas VL, Aboulafia J (1998) Activation of Ca^{2+}-activated K^+ (maxi-K^+) channel by angiotensin II in myocytes of the guinea pig ileum. Am J Physiol, 274(4 Pt 1): C983-91.

Romine MT & Anderson GF (1985) Evidence for oxytocin receptors in the urinary bladder of the rabbit. Can J Physiol Pharmacol, 63(4): 287-291.

Savaskan E (2005) The Role of the Brain Renin-Angiotensin System in neurodegenerative disorders. Current Alzheimer Research, 2(1): 29-35.

Schneider LH, Alpert J, Iversen SD (1983). CCK-8 modulation of mesolimbic dopamine: antagonism of amphetamine-stimulated behaviors. Peptides, 4: 749-753.

Seki T, Yokoshiki H, Sunagawa M, Nakamura M & Sperelakis N (1999) Angiotensin II stimulation of Ca^{2+}-channel current in vascular smooth muscle cells is inhibited by lavendustin-A and LY-294002. Pflugers Arch – Eur J Physiol, 437: 317-323.

Shimuta SI, Borges AC, Prioste RN, Paiva TB (1999) Different pathways for Ca2+ mobilization by angiotensin II and carbachol in the circular muscle of the guinea-pig ileum. Eur J Pharmacol, 367(1): 59-66.

Shokei K, Hiroshi I (2011) Molecular and Cellular Mechanisms of Angiotensin II-Mediated Cardiovascularand Renal Diseases. Pharmacol Rev, 52(1): 11-34.

Sibilia V, Pagani F, Rindi G, Lattuada N, Rapetti D, De Luca V, Campanini N, Bulgarelli I, Locatelli V, Guidobono F, Netti C (2008) Central ghrelin gastroprotection involves nitric oxide/prostaglandin cross-talk. Br J Pharmacol.,154(3): 688–697.

Sibley GNA (1984) A comparison of spontaneous and nerve-mediated activity in bladder muscle from man, pig and rabbit. J Physiol (Lond), 354: 431-443.

Siegel GJ (2006) Basic Neurochemistry, molecular, cellular and medical aspects. Burlington: Elsevier. 974 p.

Steckelings UM, Rompe F, Kaschina E, Namsolleck P, Grzesiak A, Funke-Kaiser H, Bader M, Unger T (2010) The past, present and future of angiotensin II type 2 receptor stimulation. J Renin Angiotensin Aldosterone Syst, 11(1): 67-73.

Sun Y, Asnicar M, Smith RG (2007) Central and peripheral roles of ghrelin on glucose homeostasis. Neuroendocrinology, 86(3): 215-28.

Sundler F, Aluments J, Hakanson R, Ingemansson S, Fahrenkrug J, Schaffalitzky de Muckadell OB (1977) VIP innervation of the gallbladder. Gastroenterology, 72: 1375-1377.

Swaab DF, Nijveldt F, Pool CW (1975) Distribution of oxytocin and vasopressin in the rat supraoptic and paraventricular nucleus. J Endocrinol, 67: 461-462

Szigeti GP, Somogyi GT, Csernoch L, Széll EA (2005) Age-dependence of the spontaneous activity of the rat urinary bladder. J Muscle Res Cell Motil, 26(1): 23-29.

Tack J, Depoortere I, Bisschops R, Delporte C, Coulie B, Meulemans A, Janssens J, Peeters T (2006) Infulence of ghrelin on interdigestive gastrointestinal motility in humans. Gut, 55: 327-33.

Tanabe N, Ueno A, Tsujimoto G (1993) Angiotensin II receptors in the rat urinary bladder smooth muscle: type 1 subtype receptors mediate contractile responses. J Urol, 150(3): 1056-1059.

Tanaka H, Homma K, White H, Yanagida T, Ikebe M (2008) Smooth Muscle Myosin Phosphorylated at Single Head. J Biol Chem, 283(23): 15611–15618.

Tena-Sempere M (2008) Ghrelin and reproduction: ghrelin as novel regulator of the gonadotropic axis. Vitam. Horm, 77: 285-300.

Thibonnier M, Preston JA, Dulin N, Wilkins PL, Berti-Mattera LN, Mattera R. (1997) The human V3 pituitary vasopressin receptor: ligand binding profile and density-dependent signaling pathways. Endocrinology, 138: 4109-4122

Thibonnier M (1992) Signal transduction of V1-vascular vasopressin receptors. Regul Pept, 38: 1-11

Tobin VA, Hashimoto H, Wacker DW, Takayanagi Y, Langnaese K, Caquineau C, Noack J, Landgraf R, Onaka T, Leng G, Meddle SL, Engelmann M, Ludwig M (2010) An intrinsic vasopressin system in the olfactory bulb is involved in social recognition. Nature, 464, 413-417.

Tolekova AN, Hadzhibozheva PV, Iliev RN, Georgiev TsK, Trifonova KY, Sandeva RV, Kalfin RE, Ilieva GS (2010) Participation of extracellular Ca2+) or ghrelin in peptide-mediated contraction of strips from rat urinary bladder. Regul Pept,162(1-3): 79-83.

Touyz RM, Berry C (2002) Recent advances in angiotensin II signaling. Brazilian J Med Biol Res, 35: 1001–1015.

Urata H, Kinoshita A, Misono KS, Bumpus FM, Husain A (1990) Identification of a highly specific chymase as the major angiotensin II-forming enzyme in the human heart. J Biol Chem, 265: 22348–22357.

Uvelius B, Gabella G (1998) The distribution of intramural nerves in urinary bladder after partial denervation in the female rat. Urol Res, 26: 291-297.

Uvelius B, Lundin S, Andersson KE (1990) Content and contractile effect of arginine vasopressin in rat urinary bladder. Eur J Pharmacol, 182(3): 549-554.

Vaccarino FJ, Rankin J (1989). Nucleus accumbens cholecystokinin CCK) can either attenuate or potentiate amphetamine-induced locomotor activity: evidence for rostral-caudal differences in accumbens CCK function. Behav Neurosci, 103: 831-836.

Van Der Lely AJ, Tschop M, Heiman ML, Ghigo E (2004) Biological, Physiological, Pathophysiological, and Pharmacological Aspects of Ghrelin. Endocrine Rev, 25(3): 426–457.

Van Der Lely AJ, Tschop M, Heiman ML, Ghigo E (2004) Biological, Physiological, Pathophysiological, and Pharmacological Aspects of Ghrelin. Endocrine Rev,25(3): 426–457.

Varagic J, Trask AJ, Jessup JA, Chaell MC, Ferrario CM (2008) New angiotensins. J Mol Med, 86(6): 663-671.

Vargiu R, Usai P, De Lisa, A, Argiolas A, Scarpa RM, Gessa GL, Usai E, Fraschini M, Mancinelli R (2004) Vasopressin excitatory action on smooth muscle from human renal calyx and pelvis. Pharmacol Res, 50(6): 617-622.

Vartiainen J (2009) Ghrelin, obesity and type 2 diabetes. Genetic, metabolic and epidemiological studies. Acta Univ Oul D, Oulin yliopisto, Oulu university press, Oulu, Finland, 1-114, http://herkules.oulu.fi/issn03553221

Von Bohlen, Halbach O, Albrecht D (2006) The CNS renin-angiotensin system. Cell Tissue Res.,326:599-616.

Waldeck K, Lindberg BF, Persson K, Andersson KE (1997) Characterization of angiotensin II formation in human isolated bladder by selective inhibitors of ACE and human chymase: a functional and biochemical study. Br J Pharmacol, 121(6): 1081-1086.

Wang GD, Wang XY, Hu HZ, Fang XC, Liu S, Gao N, Xia Y, Wood JD (2005) Angiotensin receptors and actions in guinea pig enteric nervous system. Am J Physiol Gastrointest Liver Physiol, 289(3): G614-26.

Watanabe T, Barker T, Berk B (2005) Angiotensin II and the Endothelium: Diverse Signals and Effects. Hypertension, 45: 163-169.

Weaver-Osterholtz D, Reams G, Wu Z, Knaus J, Campbell F, Bauer JH (1996) The urinary bladder angiotensin system: response to infusions of angiotensin I and angiotensin-converting enzyme inhibitors. Am J Kidney Dis, 28(4): 603-609.

Wiley KE, Davenport AP (2002) Comparioson of vasodilators in human internal mammary artery: ghrelin is a potent physiological antagonist of endothelin-1. Br J Pharmacol, 136(8): 1146-1152.

Xu D, Yu BP, Luo HS, Chen LD (2008) Control of gallbladder contractions by cholecystokinin through cholecystokinin-A receptors on gallbladder interstitial cells of Cajal. World J Gastroenterol 141(8): 2882-2887.

Yamada S, Takeuchi C, Oyunzul L, Ito Y (2009). Bladder angiotensin-II receptors: characterization and alteration in bladder outlet obstruction. Eur Urol, 55(2): 482-489.

Yankov K (2006) System Identification of Biological Processes. Proc. 20-th Int.Conf. "Systems for Automation of Engineering and Research SAER-2006. Varna, Bulgaria, 144-149.

Yankov K (2009) Recognition and function association of experimental data. Proc. of the Int. Conference on Information Technologies InfoTech-2009, Varna, Bulgaria, 131-141.

Yankov K. (2010) Preprocessing of Experimental Data in Korelia Software. Trakia Journal of Sciences, 83): 41-48.

Yankov K (2011) Evaluation of characteristic parameters of dynamic models. Proceedings of the International Conference on Information Technologies InfoTech-2011,15th – 17 September 2011, Bulgaria, http://www.tu-sofia.bg/saer/index.html.

Yannielli P, Molyneux P, Harrington M, Golombek D (2007) Ghrelin Effects on the Circadian System of Mice. The Journal of Neuroscience, 271(1): 2890 –2895.

Zelena D, Mergl Z, Makara GB (2006) The role of vasopressin in diabetes mellitus-induced hypothalamo-pituitary-adrenal axis activation: studies in Brattleboro rats.Brain Res Bull.,69(1):48-56.

Zetler G (1983) Neuroleptic-like effects of ceruletide and cholecystokinin octapeptide: interactions with apomorphine, methyphenidate and picrotoxin. Eur J Pharmacol 94, 261-270.

Zhang J, Ritter RC (2012) Circulating GLP-1 and CCK-8 reduce food intake by capsaicin-insensitive, nonvagal mechanisms. Am J Physiol Regul Integr Comp Physiol 302(2): R264-R273.

Chapter 7

Effect of Cadmium Contaminated Diet in Controlling Water Behavior by *Meriones shawi*

Sihem Mbarek, Tounes Saidi and Rafika Ben Chaouacha-Chekir

Additional information is available at the end of the chapter

http://dx.doi.org/10.5772/50421

1. Introduction

Body fluid regulation is highly diverse among different animals according to their phylogenic position and the ecological condition [1]. The maintenance of water homeostasis in arid and semi-arid rodent habitats is a critical body function to survive the continually changing environmental condition. The combined effects of anatomical adaptations, behavioural patterns and interactions between hormonal systems allow these small mammals to minimize energetic costs and to finely balance body fluids under a wide range of conditions [2-3]. This is made possible essentially, by homeostatic mechanisms that concentrate urine as an indicator of water regulation efficiency as well as an advantage for colonization and survival [4].

Meriones shawi (Muridae) a semi-desert rodent found in the coastal zone of North-west Africa from Morocco to Egypt [5], has a particular ability to support water restriction until several months [6]. It appears that water intake and water loss are finely balanced by *Meriones shawi*. Water intake was provided from preformed water of food and by metabolic water production as described by King and Bradshaw [7]. Water loss was limited by the production of very dry feces. In addition, *Meriones shawi* produces concentrated urines as results of high plasma concentrations of arginine-vaspressin (AVP) and a large capacity of increasing hypothalamic AVP synthesis and hypophyseal storage [8]. The mean value to concentrate urine in the *Meriones shawi* submitted to water dehydration during 10 days, increased from 1500 mOsm $Kg^{-1}H_20$/ to 3000 mOsm.Kg^{-1} H_20 under laboratory conditions. The maximal capacity to concentrate urine (recorded under laboratory conditions) ranged from approximately 4500 mOsm Kg^{-1} H_20 in the *Meriones shawi* [9]. The alterations of kidney Na-K-ATPase activity, including pronounced heterogeneity of ATPase distributions in nephrons and increased Na-K-ATPase activity in the medullary limb, observed in response to water restriction, can be responsible for this ability [10]. However, AVP is the most important hormone to elaborate urines largely hyperosmotic to plasma. A comparative study of water controlling behavior was done between rat laboratory and *Meriones shawi* demonstrated that the level of AVP is 4-fold greater than in dehydrated rats [11]. AVP levels are highly dependent on the state of hydration and correlate with urinary osmolality [12].

AVP or antidiuretic hormone (ADH), is known to be primarily involved in water absorption in the distal nephron of the kidney in mammals. This peptide is synthesized in the soma of hypothalamic magnocellular neurosecretory cells (MNCSs) located in supraoptic (SON) and paraventricular (PVN) nuclei. After water deprivation the axons MNCs project to the neurohypophysis, where Ca^{2+} dependent exocytosis in their nerve terminals causes the release of AVP in blood circulation. The small peptide is secreted by the neurohypophysis in response to increases in plasma osmolality. AVP effects on the renal tubule are mediated by hormone binding to V2 type basolateral receptors coupled trough Gs to adenylyl cyclase and activation of the cyclic adenosine monophosphate - Protein kinase A (cAMP-PKA) cascade [13]. The hydroosmotic action causes a dramatic increase in the osmotic water permeability of connecting cells, principal cells and inner medullary collecting duct cells. The result is highly concentrated urines produced in response to water restriction.

The success of rodent to survive harsh environment condition goes back to several years ago. However, these animals are faced to substantial anthropogenic threats due to the introduction of heavy metals in environment in the last decades. Cadmium (Cd), a nonessential heavy metal, is widely distributed in the environment due to its use in primary metal industries and phosphate fertilizers [15, 16]. Food and cigarette smoke are the biggest sources of Cd exposure for the general population [17]. In humans, Cd exposure leads to a variety of adverse effects and contributes to the development of serious pathological conditions [18-19] linked to enhanced aging process as well as cancer [20-21]. Cd produces also neurotoxicity with a complex pathology [22-23]. In animals, Cd was shown to be toxic to all tissues such as liver [24], reproductive organs including the placenta, testis and ovaries [17, 25]. Several studies in some industrial sites in Tunisia showed that some habitats of *Meriones shawi* became contaminated by Cd [26-27] *Meriones shawi* have accumulated cadmium on different organs particularly on kidney and liver. It has been reported that kidneys, which play a major role in hydro-mineral maintenance, are considered to be the organ that is most sensitive to Cd, depending on exposure dose, time and administration route [28]. Several studies indicated that the main critical effect of cadmium exposure is kidney dysfunction. Excretion of low molecular weight proteins is characteristic of damage to the proximal tubules of the kidney. The increased excretion of low-molecular weight proteins in the urine is a result of proximal tubular cell damage [29]. This raises the possibility that body fluid homeostasis and vasopressinergic system could be subtly disrupted by Cd exposure. In this study, we were interested to determine whether Cd naturally incorporated in food would alter the water balance in *Meriones shawi* who appears to show a remarkable physiology flexibility of water regulation in both time and space. Effects of Cd exposure upon the water-conserving abilities of this specie were assessed through measurements of water metabolism (total body water (TBW), water influx (Fin), water efflux (Fout) and water turnover rates (WTR) under differing water availabilities. Water fluxes were determined by direct analysis following the principles described by Holleman and Dieterich [30]. Cd effects in the brain were also determined by immunohistochemistry in the supraoptic (SON) and paraventricular (PVN) nuclei at the control level of the central AVP which is the most important hormone in the regulation of water balance in mammals.

2. Material and methods

2.1. Animals and housing conditions

All experiments were carried out on adult male of Muridae; *Meriones shawi* [31] originating from the south of Tunisia. The rodents were captured from non-polluted regions and kept in captivity in our breeding facility for two generations. The animals were put in single cages and housed in an air-conditioned room maintained at 25 ± 1°C at a relative humidity of 45 ± 10 %, with a 12 h dark-light cycle. The diet of the control group consisted of granular flour mixed with distilled water at the dose of 1 L /1.5 Kg of granular flour. Contaminated diets of treated animals consisted of granule flour mixed with a solution of cadmium chloride ($CdCl_2$) at dose (1 g Cd/1L H_2O/1.5 kg of granule flour) [32]. Food was given in the form of balls dried at 60 ° C for 72 hours. Water was supplied *ad libitum*.

Animals were randomly selected and divided into four groups. Eight animals, the first goup was used as control (C). Water was given *ad libitum*. Meriones of the second group (8 animals) received the same diet but were deprived of water (D-). The third group was treated with Cd in the form of $CdCl_2$ (Cd) at dose (1 g Cd/1L H_2O/1.5 kg of granule flour). The last group was also treated with $CdCl_2$ at the same dose but was deprived water D+Cd.

For immunohistochemistry study, treatment period had lasted from eight days to two weeks. Each animal was put in a metabolic cage for eight days in order to collect feces and 24 h urine each day at the same time. Urine samples were collected on paraffin oil to prevent evaporation and measured in mL/day. Daily consumption of drinking water and food of each group were measured throughout the study. It was not possible to collect urine since the 10 days of dehydration.

All of the protocols were carried out in accordance with French standard ethical guidelines for laboratory animals (agreement 75-178, 5_16_2000).

2.2. Techniques

Body weight of each animal was determined throughout the experiment. Blood samples were collected from the infra-orbital sinus into heparinized hematocrit capillary tubes, immediately before the experimental period and eight days later. These samples were centrifuged at 1500 g x for 10 min in order to determine hematocrit. At the end of experimentation rodents were sacrificed by decapitation, and brain, kidneys and livers were immediately removed and weighed. The weight of organs (%) was calculated as g /100 g of body weight. Finally these organs were dried at 60° C and weighed for the determination of dry weight.

2.3. Determination of water fluxes

Water fluxes were determined by direct analysis following the principles described by Holleman and Dieterich [30]. Rates of water flux represent the loss of water via excretion and evaporation and the simultaneous input of water, via metabolic water production and pre-formed water via food and drink (Nagy and Costa 1980). Free water content of the food determined by drying to constant weight at 60 °C was 3 %. The metabolic water content was determined from carbohydrate, fat and protein composition [33]. Thus 1 g of given food contains 0.509 mL of water. The intact unshaven carcasses were sublimated to dryness. The difference between live and dry weight was taken as total body water (TBW).

After determining urine volume and feces weight, urine samples were frozen at -30 °C while the feces were dried for 72 h. Water efflux was calculated as the difference between the influx and total body water. Water fluxes are expressed in H_2O mL per day. Finally these fluxes were normalized to the average body weights and expressed in $kg^{-0.82}$. In small mammals an allometric relationship exists between the water efflux or influx and body weight (W) in kilograms, which is $Fin=K.W^{0.82}$ ([34-35], expressed as mL/day/100 g body weight.

2.4. Tissue preparation

Meriones were anesthetized with sodium pentobarbital (70 mg/kg, i.p; Sanofi, Libourne,France) and perfused transcardially with heparin in physiological saline, followed by 500 mL of a freshly prepared solution of 4 % (wt / vol) paraformaldehyde in phosphate – buffered saline (PBS ; pH = 7.4). The brains were rapidly removed and postfixed overnight in 4 % paraformaldehyde at 4 °C. Forty micrometer thick coronal sections were cut with a Vibratome (VT 1000S; Leica, Nussloch, Germany). Brain sections were collected in cold PBS.

2.5. Immunohistochemistry

Free-floating sections were pretreated for 20 min with 3 % hydrogen peroxide in PBS to quench endogenous peroxidase. They were then washed with PBS (3 x 10 min), preincubated for 90 min at room temperature in PBS containing 0.05 %. Triton X-100 and 3 % normal horse serum. Sections were incubated for 36 h at 4 °C with Mouse anti-AVP antibody (1: 5000 dilution).

After incubation, sections were rinsed extensively with PBS (four times, 15 min) and incubated for 1.5 h in a 1/100 dilution of biotin conjugated horse anti-goat antibody and other secondary antibodies. Texas Red conjugated rabbit anti-mouse antibody (1/200; dilution; Jackson ImmunoResearch). For amplification, we used tyramide signal amplification fluorescence system technology (NEN, Boston, MA, USA). For details see Banisadr et al. [36]. After washing, sections were mounted onto gelatin-coated slides in Vectashield (Vector) and observed on fluorescent microscope (BX61; Olympus, Melville, NY) and a connected image-acquisition software (Analysis) was used.

2.6. Statistical analysis

Data are shown as the mean ± SEM. All results were compared to control animals (C), as well as to the Cd-exposed animals (Cd). For all our experiment, a two-way ANOVA was used to analyze the differences between groups, followed by a Dunnett's test with a threshold of significance of $p < 0.05$ and $p < 0.01$ to detect specific differences, using a statistical software package (XLSTAT version 2009.1.1).

3. Results

3.1. Body mass

During the eight days of experimentation, body mass doesn't change significantly in the control group. Body weight loss represented 5.77 ± 0.05 % in *Meriones* treated with Cd (expressed in % of initial body weight). A higher significant increase in body weight loss (16 ± 0.19 % of initial body weight) was observed following 8 days of water restriction. The body weight loss (19.34 ± 0.29 %) is greater in the *Meriones* group both water-deprived and treated with Cd.

3.2. Relative weights of organs

Relative weight of liver in controls is an average of 0.05 ± 0.01. Cd exposure significantly altered the relative weight of liver (0.036 ± 0.01) following eight days of treatment. Water restriction had no effect on relative weight of liver as compared to control *Meriones*.

Decrease in relative weight of liver was also observed in water-deprived group and simultaneously treated with Cd. No differences were found in relative kidney weights (6.8 ± 0.9) in all groups under all experimental conditions.

3.3. Food consumption

Consumption of food was expressed per 100 g of body weight. Control animals consumed an average of 4.5 g/day of food. There was a significant ($p < 0.01$) decrease of food intake in the Cd-exposed group (2.54 ± 0.2 g daily). Food intake of the water deprived groups was similar to that of the controls. When water deprivation was combined with Cd exposure, the decrease in food intake became larger and statistically significant compared with both control ($p < 0.01$) and Cd-exposed groups ($p<0.05$).

3.4. Hematocrit

After eight days of experimentation, hematocrit (44.32 ± 1.08 %) did not change significantly in any treatment condition as compared to day 1 (Fig. 3).

3.5. Water metabolism

Water metabolism data are shown in Table 1.

Treatment	Initial body weight (g)	Total body water (mL)	Total body water (%W)	Water influx mL	Water efflux mL	Water influx ml $Kg^{-0.82} d^{-1}$	Water efflux mL.$Kg^{-0.82} d^{-1}$	WTR in (% body water d^{-1})	WTR out (% body water d^{-1})	Urinary osmolality mOs/kg H_20	Plasma osmolality (mOs/kg H_20)
Control	117.44 ±3.66	62.97 ±2.55	55.79 ±2.74	10.90 ±3.63	10.27 ±3.66	63.83 ±22.70	60.16 ±22.79	17.36 ±6.44	16.37 ±6.43	1100 ± 2	307.6 ± 4.2
Cd-exposed Meriones	134.41 ±19.37	61.09 ±5.28	48.38 ±5.87	10.04 ±3.08	9.34 ±3.04	50.50 ±11.12	47.11 ±11.53	15.51 ±4.55	14.43 ±4.52	1600 ± 1.9**	332 ± 3
Deprived water Meriones	120.37 ±16.85	64.89 ±1.23	61.30 ±9.28	•• ** 2.17 ±0.23	•• ** 1.93 ±0.56	• ** 12.48 ±1.27	• ** 11.96 ±3.34	•• ** 3.18 ±1.06	•• ** 3.12 ±0.67	•• ** 1700 ±1.9	345 ± 3
Deprived water and Cd-exposed Meriones	128.25 ±18.67	67.59 ±1.36	60.50 ±9.99	•• ** 1.73 ±0.50	•• ** 1.81 ±0.76	• ** 9.32 ±2.11	• ** 9.62 ±3.28	•• ** 2.45 ±0.73	•• ** 2.66 ±1.09	•• ** 1162 ±2	307.6 ± 4.2

Table 1. Effects of Cd exposure on water metabolism (Total Body Water, Water influx, Water efflux, and Water Turnover Rates (WTR)and urinary and plasma osmolalities) in adult *Meriones shawi* male under hydrated or deprived water conditions. Data are expressed as mean ± SEM from 6 animals in each group.** p <0.01significantly different from controls C.• p<0.05; ••p<0.01 signifficantly different from Cd-exposed Meriones.

Total body water content in control group was 55.79 ± 2.74 (expressed by % of body weight). Throughout the experiments, body water was not significantly altered in any group. In animals having free access to water, water enters through metabolic water production and pre-formed water via food and drink.

The value of water influx was 10.90 ± 3.63 ml/ 63.83 ± 22.79 ml.$Kg^{-0.82}$ .d^{-1}. This water influx (Fin) was not significantly affected in the group treated with Cd in comparison to control group. The loss of water via excretion (urine and fecal) and evaporation was Fout =10.27 ± 3.66 ml/60.16 22.79 ml.$kg^{-0.82}$.d-1. Water fluxes rate were equal (Fin = Fout). This indicates that animals were in water equilibrium. After, one week of Cd exposure, water flux rates were not significantly affected in the group treated with Cd in comparison to control group and water equilibrium was maintained throughout the experiment.

Following one week of dehydration, the water influx rates was significantly decreased from about 5 times in Meriones treated or not with Cd ($p<0.01$). Cd exposure may not affected the water intake during our experiment.

In spite variations in water intake in different experimental conditions, all animals were in water equilibrium where water influx (Fin) and efflux (Fout) rates were equal (Fin = Fout).

3.6. Distribution of immunohistochemical staining for AVP

In control *Meriones shawi*, AVP immunostaining was found to be homogeneously distributed in the large magnocellular neurons of SON (Fig. 2) and PVN (Fig. 3). In agreement with previous, in the absence of Cd ingestion, there was a significant compensatory increase in AVP immunostaining by the SON of deprived animals following eight days of water restriction (Fig. 2C) and two weeks (Fig. 2D) compared to controls animals (fig 2A and B). This increase in AVP immunostaining was also observed in PVN respectively after eight days and two weeks of water restriction (Fig. 3C) and (Fig. 3D) compared respectively to controls animals (fig 3a and B).

Similarly to what was observed for AVP immunostaining in deprived animals without Cd, AVP immunoreactivity is strongly increased in SON following eight days of water restriction (Fig. 2E) and PVN (Fig. 2F) compared to controls animals respectively (Fig.2A) and (Fig.3A). The increase of AVP immunostaining became more important by prolonged experiment for two weeks respectively in SON (Fig. 2F) and PVN (Fig. 3F).

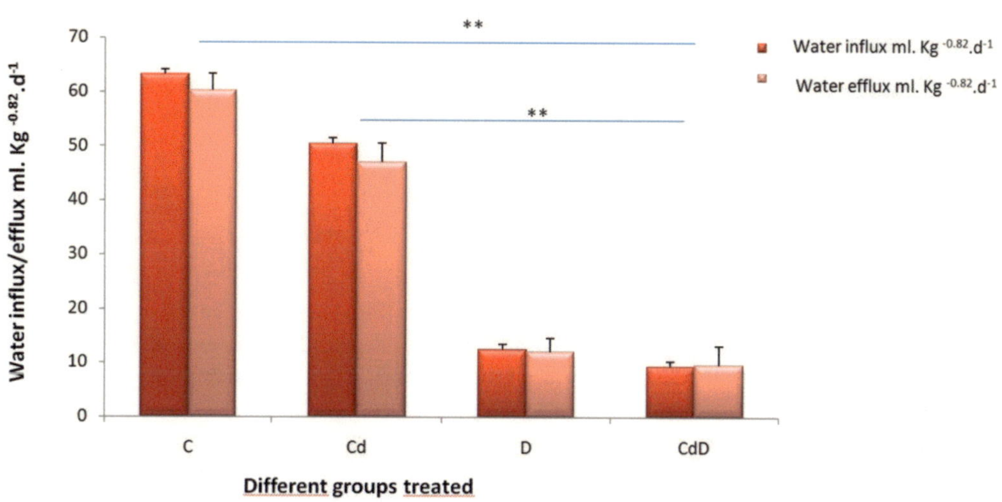

Figure 1. Effects of Cd exposure on water Water influx and efflux in adult *Meriones shawi* male under hydrated or deprived water conditions. Data are expressed as mean ± SEM from 6 animals in each group.

However, AVP immunostaining from deprived water animals in the presence of Cd was markedly and significantly lower in SON (Fig. 2G) than in deprived water animals but not treated with Cd for a week (Fig. 2C). This decrease of AVP immunostaining becomes more important following two weeks of treatment (Fig. 2H) in comparison in two weeks deprived water animals not treated with Cd (Fig. 2D). Similar effect of AVP depletion in SON was also observed in PVN in simultaneously deprived water group and Cd-exposed Meriones during eight days (Fig. 3G) and two weeks (Fig. 3H) in comparison to those eight days deprived water group and two weeks deprived water groups and not treated with Cd.

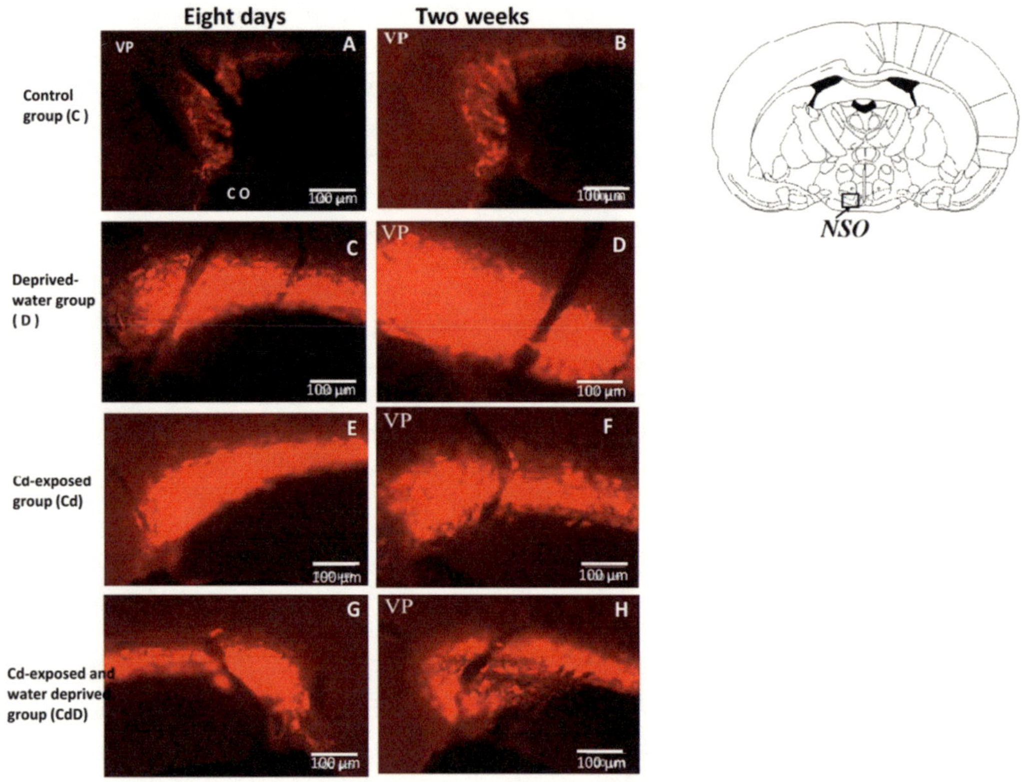

Figure 2. Effect of Cd exposure on AVP immunoreactivity distribution in the hypothalamic supraoptic nuclei (NSO) in *Meriones shawi.* Control group (A,B) , eight days deprived-water group (C), two weeks deprived-water group (D), Eight days Cd-exposed group E, two weeks Cd-exposed group (F), 8 days Cd-exposed and also deprived water group (G), two weeks Cd-exposed and also deprived water group (H).Water deprivation increased the immunohistochemical signal in SON nuclei (C); this increase became more important following two weeks of water deprivation (D) . Similar effect was observed when Meriones are exposed to Cd following one week (E) and two weeks (F). However, Exposure to Cd causes a decrease in immunoreactivity of vasopressin at SON by Meriones deprived water for a week (G) compared to those water deprived group but not treated with Cd (C). This decrease was also observed after two weeks of treatment (H) as compared to water deprived Meriones (D). Scale bars =100 µm.

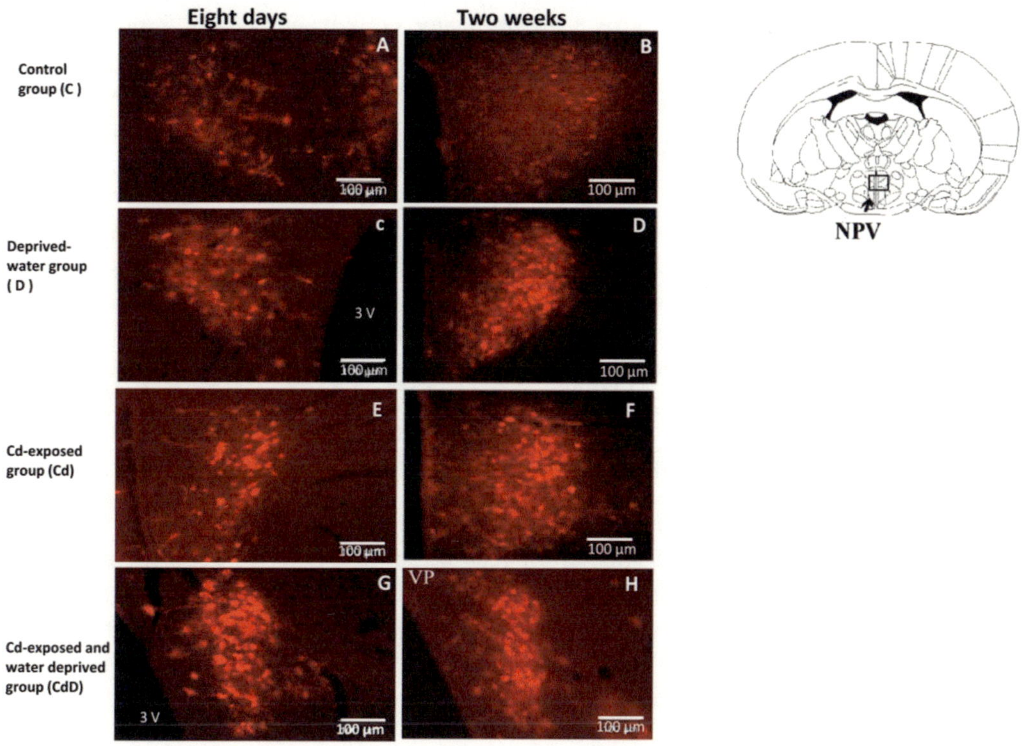

Figure 3. Effect of Cd exposure on AVP immunoreactivity distribution in the hypothalamic paraventricular nuclei (NPV) in *Meriones shawi*. Control group (A,B) , eight days deprived-water group (C), two weeks deprived-water group (D), Eight days Cd-exposed group E, two weeks Cd-exposed group (F), 8 days Cd-exposed and also deprived water group (G), two weeks Cd-exposed and also deprived water group (H).Water deprivation increased the immunohistochemical signal in NPV nuclei (C); this increase became more important following two weeks of water deprivation (D) . Similar effect was observed when Meriones are exposed to Cd following one week (E) and two weeks (F). However, Exposure to Cd causes a decrease in immunoreactivity of vasopressin at NPV by Meriones deprived water for a week (G) compared to those water deprived group but not treated with Cd (C). This decrease was also observed after two weeks of treatment (H) as compared to water deprived Meriones (D). Scale bars =100 µm.

3.7. Effect of Cd on water metabolism

Meriones shawi, success dry and wet seasons by stimulating anti-diuretic and diuretic systems alternately. The maintenance of tonicity of body fluids by within a very narrow physiological range is made possible by well-developed homeostatic mechanisms that control the intake and loss of water [2, 37]. This capacity was also observed when *Meriones shawi* was treated with Cd under various conditions of water deprivation. *Meriones shawi* are able to maintain body water (55.79 %) status under water deprivation conditions. The absence of change in hematocrit value observed by deprived water groups treated or not with Cd (45%) suggests that regulatory processes occur, resulting in the maintenance of body water content and increase in urine concentration [38-39]. Whether in nature or under laboratory conditions, control groups were in water equilibrium (water influx = water efflux) [32]. The value of water influx was 10.90 ± 3.63 ml/ 63.83 ± 22.79 $ml.Kg^{-0.82}.d^{-1}$ (figure 1). This water influx (Fin) was not significantly affected in the group treated with Cd in comparison to control group. The loss of water via excretion (urine and fecal) and evaporation was Fout =10.27 ± 3.66 ml./60.16 ± 22.79 $ml.kg^{-0.82}.d^{-1}$. Water fluxes rate were equal (Fin = Fout). This indicates that animals were in water equilibrium. After, one week of Cd exposure, water flux rates were not significantly affected in the group treated with Cd in comparison to control group and water equilibrium was maintained throughout the experiment. Following one week of dehydration, the water influx rates was significantly decreased from about 5 times in Meriones treated or not with Cd ($p<0.01$). Cd exposure appears not to impair this capacity during our experiment. However in water deprived animals there was a lower rate of water influx and efflux compared to controls. This low rate of water influx and efflux was similar in water deprived animals and treated with Cd simultaneously (water metabolism are shown in table 1).

The urinary osmolality (UO) in the control *Meriones* group was around 1100 $mOsm.Kg^{-1}.H_20$. The mean value increased significantly from 1100 mOsm $Kg^{-1}H_20$/ to 1600 $mOsm.Kg^{-1}$ H_20 following one week of water restriction. This value not change when animals were exposed to Cd [40]. The plasma osmolality (PO) was around 270 $mOsm.Kg^{-1}$. It was not changed in all groups following one and two weeks of experiment. Hematocrit was around (44.32 ± 1.08 %). It did not change in any treatment condition as compared to day 1. All these results are shown in table 1.

In spite of the variations in water metabolism, all animals were in water equilibrium, at the end of experimentation. All these results indicate that even under the most stringent conditions *Meriones shawi* has a strong capacity to maintain a homeostasis state. It seems evident that water restriction induced a pronounced body mass loss in animals after eight days of treatment without available drinking water. This indicates a depletion of reserves of endogenous metabolic water supplies as an alternative to fresh water [9]. Although changes in body mass in Cd-exposed animals are assumed to be due to reduction of daily consumption of food, this decrease of food uptake became larger in animals both deprived water and treated with Cd. This is in agreement with the findings of Pettersen et al. [41] who demonstrated that rats exposed to Cd become anorexic. An important finding in this study, described by other authors Woltowski et al. [42] and Leffel et al. [43] was the early occurrence of Cd induced hepatic damage manifested by lower liver weight, which was explained by the high level of Cd found in livers of exposed animals. As shown by Sudo et al. [44] Cd preferentially localizes in hepatocytes after administration, and its concentration may exceed the capacity of intracellular constituents, mainly metallothioneins (MTs) to bind Cd [45]. MT-bound Cd then appears in the blood plasma [44] and is efficiently filtered through the glomeruli, and subsequently taken up by the tubules leading to its accumulation in kidney [46-47].

In order to maintain physiological serum osmolality, water intake and water loss are finely balanced by *Meriones shawi* even under water restriction and Cd exposure condition (fig 1). It appears that *Meriones shawi* are able to retain water by excretion of highly concentrated urine [8]. Water loss was also limited by the lowered faecal water loss achieved by the production of very dry feces. In deprived water Meriones we show that water intake was provided from preformed water of food and by metabolic water production as described by Speakman [48] and King and Bradshaw [49]. Our findings are in agreement with previous reports showing that renal concentrating mechanisms are the first line of defense against water depletion [4, 12, 50]. It is well established that modifications of serum osmolality during depletion are detected via osmoreceptors by magnocellular mainly located in the hypothalamic supraoptic nucleus (SON) and paraventricular nucleus (PVN) in the brain [39, 51]. These neurons increase their electrophysiological activity during water restriction leading to an increase of AVP synthesis [52- 53] (and facilitates sustained antidiuresis [54] (De Mota et al. 2004). In contrast to what was observed in the laboratory rat where dehydration causes a dramatic depletion of hypothalamic AVP immunoreactivity in both SON and PVN [55- 56], water restriction induced in our model an increase in expression of AVP. This increase becomes more important with time of restriction water.

Interestingly, the ability of acute systemic dehydration to produce AVP in both SON and PVN in *Meriones shawi* deprived water and not treated with Cd, was also observed while treating Meriones with Cd but not deprived water. We hypothesized that potential effects of Cd might include exaggerated synthesis of AVP during Cd exposure in our model *Meriones shawi* and support the idea of an increase of AVP as result of Cd intoxication (see figure 2 and 3). These findings suggest that Cd ingestion has potential effects on the vasopressinergic system that responds with elevated synthesis of AVP under stimulated conditions [57]. A large number of studies have demonstrated that Cd exposure produce marked neuroendocrine changes in animals [58- 59] and human [60].

The current study is the first to explore the potential impact of Cd exposure on the magnocellular neuroendocrine system responsible for hydromineral balance. In this paper, we shown an involvement of the hypothalamo-vasopressinergic system of AVP, wish plays a fundamental role in the maintenance of body fluid homeostasis, in the protective reactions of the organism during Cd exposure in *Meriones shawi* by secreting arginine-vasopressin in response to a variety of physiological stimuli, including osmotic [61-63] and nonosmotic stimuli [64, 65]. In support of this, we found that water metabolism was identical in both groups of deprived water *Meriones* and treated *Meriones* with Cd respectively. In contrast, the adaptive response of vasopressin enhancement secretion in both SON and PVN under stimulated conditions as dehydration or Cd exposure in *Meriones shawi,* was attenuated in Meriones simultaneously exposed to Cd and dehydration of water, as compared to deprived water but not treated with Cd group. Our results show an inhibitory effect of Cd exposure on AVP immunoreactivity in both SON and PVN in response to acute water restriction in adult male *Meriones.* We hypothesized that potential effects of Cd might modifies vasopressinergic system which is amplified under water restriction, where AVP neurons are under constant stimulation and suggested that vasopressinergic system is subtly disrupted. Similar effect of AVP depletion in both SON and PVN, produced by Cd ingestion in deprived water was also observed in deprived water laboratory rats treated by an organochlorine pollutant (polychlorinated biphenyls (PCBs) during 15 days [66]. According to these authors, the AVP decline was attributable to specific effects of overt toxicity and/or malaise oral of PCBs on vasopressinergic hypothalamic cells function. In combination with the efficacy of *in vitro* application, these data are consistent with direct actions on components of the hypothalamo-neurohypophysial system present within the SON [67-68]. PCBs has been reported to inhibit nitric oxide synthase activity. It is noteworthy that the inhibition of nitric oxide production in SON tissue punches produces a virtually identical, selective effect on dehydration stimulated intranuclear AVP release *in vitro* [69] and has been reported to exaggerate pituitary depletion of AVP in the intact deprived water rat [70] .

Most strikingly, vasopressin is recognized as circulating hormone. Its actions were essentially confined to peripheral organs. However, currently AVP have been shown to be released in the brain as chemical messengers. AVP, like many peptides, when released within the brain, plays an important role in social behaviour. In rats, AVP is implicated in paternal behaviors, such as grooming, crouching over and contacting pups. AVP is also important for partner preference and pair bonding, particularly for males in a variety of species. It has been shown that AVP has powerful influences on complex behaviours [71]. Disruption of vasopressinergic system has been linked to several neurobehavioural disorders including prader-Willi syndrome, affective disorders, obsessive-compulsive disorder and polymorphisms of V1a vasopressin receptor have been linked to autism [72].

4. Conclusion

On the basis of the current study, we conclude that Cd exposure modifies the vasopressinergic neuronal system and provides information regarding the neurotoxicity risks that this element presents for mammals and human populations exposed to Cd even to low amounts without affecting directly water metabolism. We are currently trying to study the linkage between Cd exposure and water controlling behavior at different level of the central nervous system.

Author details

Sihem Mbarek*, Tounes Saidi and Rafika Ben Chaouacha-Chekir
Laboratory of Ecophysiology and Food Processes,
Higher Institute of Biotechnology at Sidi Thabet Ariana, University of Manouba, Tunisia

5. References

[1] Willmer P, Stone G, Johnston IM. Environmental Physiology of Animals. Blackwell Science, Oxford 2000.

* Corresponding Author

[2] Nagy KA. Water economy of free-living desert animals. Int Cong series 2004; 1275: 291-297.

[3] Elgot A, Ahboucha S, Bouyatas MM, Montange MF, Gamrani H. Water deprivation affects serotoninergic system and glycoprotein secretion in the sub-commissural organ of a desert rodent *Meriones shawi*. Neurosci. Lett. 2009; 466: 6-10.

[4] Bozinovic F, Gallardo P. The water economy of South American desert rodents: From integrative to molecular physiological ecology Review. Comp. Biochem. Physiol. C. Toxicol. Pharmacol 2006; 142(3-4):163-72.

[5] Corbet GB. The Mammals of the Palaearctic Region: a Taxonomic Review. British Museum (Natural History), Cornell University Press. 1978.

[6] Gamrani H, ElgoA. El Hiba O, Fèvre –Montange M. Cellular plasticity in the supraoptic and paraventricular nuclei after prolonged dehydration in the desert rodent *Meriones shawi*: Vasopressin and GFAP immunohistochemical study *Brain. Res.* 2011; 1375: 85-92.

[7] King JM, Bradshaw SD. Comparative water metabolism of Barrow Island macropodid marsupials: Hormonal *versus* behavioural-dependent mechanisms of body water conservation. Gen Comp Endocrinology 2008; 155 (2):378-385.

[8] Rabhi M, Ugrumov MV, Goncharevskaya OA, Bengelloun W, Calas A, Natochin YV. Development of the hypothalamic vasopressin system and nephrons in *Meriones shawi* during ontogenesis. Anat Embryol (Berl). 1996; 193 (3): 281-296.

[9] Ben Chaouacha-Chekir R. *Fonction thyroidienne et métabolisme hydrique chez quelques gerbillidés du sud tunisien.* 1989Thèse doct. d'état. Museum National d'Histoire naturelle et Université Pierre et Marie Curie, Paris 6.

[10] Doucet A, Barlet C, and Baddouri K. Effect of water intake on Na-K-ATPase in nephron segments of the desert rodent, *Jaculus orientalis. Pflugers Arch.* 1987; 408: 129–132

[11] Sellami A, Maurel D, Kosa A , Sicud P. Réponses hormonales du mérion, un rongeur désertique à la privation d'eau prolongée : comparaison avec le rat. Mésogée 2005 ; 61 : 1-17.

[12] Baddouri K, Butlen D, Imbert-Teboul, M, Le Bouffant F, Marchetti J, Chabardes D, and Morel F. Plasma antidiuretic hormone levels and kidney responsiveness to vasopressin in the jerboa. *Jaculus orientalis. Gen. Comp. Endocrinol.* 1984; 54 : 203–215.

[13] Birnbaumer, M Seiblod A Gilbert S Ishido M Barberis C Antaramian A Brabet P Roesnthal W. Molecular cloning of the receptor for human antidiuretic hormone. Nature 1992; 357, 333-335.

[14] Ben Chaouacha-chekir R, Leloup J, Lachiver F. Influence of thyroid status on water metabolism and survival of normal and deprived water desert rodents *Meriones libycus*. Gen Comp Endocrinol 1997; 105:1-8.

[15] Morselt AFW. Environmental pollutants and disease. Toxicology 1991; 70: 1-132.

[16] Novelli ELB, Vieira EP, Rodrigues NL, Rribas B. Risk Assessment of Cadmium Toxicity on Hepatic and Renal Tissues of Rats. Environ Res. 1998 *A* 79: 102-105.

[17] Waalkes MP, Coogan TP, Barter RA. Toxicological Principles of Metal Carcinogenesis with Special Emphasis on Cadmium. Critical Rev in Toxicol 1992, 22 (3-4): 175-201.

[18] Bernard A.Renal dysfunction induced by cadmium: biomarkers of critical effects. Biometals 2004; 17 (5):519-523.

[19] Jin T, Nordberg G, Ye Tingting, BO M, Wang H, Zhu G, Kong Q, Bernard A. Osteoporosis and renal dysfunction in a general population exposed to cadmium in China. Environ Res 2004; 96: 353-369.

[20] Waalkes MP. Cadmium carcinogenesis. Mutat Res 2003; 533 (1-2):107-120.

[21] Huff J, Lunn RM, Waalkes MP, Tomatis L, Infante PF Cadmium-induced cancers in animals and in humans. Int J Occup Environ Health. 2007; 13(2):202-212.

[22] Shukla GS, Singhal RL.The present status of biological effects of toxic metals in the environment : lead, cadmium, and manganese. Can J Physiol Pharmacol 1984; 62: 1015-1031.

[23] Gupta A, Gupta A, Murthy RC, Chandra SV. Neurochemical changes in developing rat brain after pre- and postnatal cadmium exposure. Bull Environ Contam Toxicol 1993; 51:12-17.

[24] Newairy AA, El-Sharaky AS, Badreldeen MM, Eweda SM, Sheweita SA. The hepatoprotective effects of selenium against cadmium toxicity in rats. Toxicology 2007; 242(1-3):23-30.

[25] Leffel EK, Wolf C, Poklis A, White Jr. KL. Drinking water exposure to cadmium, an environmental contaminant, results in the exacerbation of autoimmune disease in the murine model. Toxicology 2003; 188: 233-250.

[26] Messaoudi I, Ben Chaouacha-chekir R. Fixation du cadmium (Cd) par différents tissus et ses effets sur le poids corporel et la calcémie chez un rongeur, Gerbillidé, *Meriones shawi shawi*. Mammalia 2002; t 66 (4) : 553-562.

[27] Sebei A, chaabani F, Ouerfelli MK, Abdeljaoued S. Evaluation de la contamination des sols par des métaux lourds dans la région minière de Fedj Lahdhoum (NW de la Tunisie). Revue Méditérranéenne de L'Environnement 2006 ; 1-12.

[28] Yasuda M, Miwa A, Kitagawa M. Morphotometric studies of renal lesions in Itai-Itai disease : Chronic cadmium nephropathy. Nephron 1995; 69: 14-19.

[29] Ikeda M, Ezaki T, Tsukahara T, Moriguchi J, Furuki K, Fukui Y, Ukai SH, Sakurai H. Critical evaluation of alpha1- and beta2-microglobulins in urine as markers of cadmium-induced tubular dysfunction. *Biometals* 2004; 17: 539-541.

[30] Holleman DF, Dietrich RA. Body water content and turnover in several species of rodents as evaluated by the tritiated water method. J Mamm. 1973; 54: 456-465.

[31] Nicol SC. Rates of water turnover in Marsupials and Eutheriens: a comparative review with new data on the Tasmanian Devil. Austr J Zool 1978; 26: 465-473.

[32] Chevret P, Dobigny G. Systematics and evolution of the subfamily Gerbillinae (Mammalia, Rodentia, Muridae). Mol Phylogenetics Evol 2005; 35:674-688.

[33] Mbarek S., Saidi T., Ben Mansour H., Rostene W., Parsadaniantz S.M., Ben Chaouacha-chekir R. Effect of cadmium on water metabolism regulation by *Meriones shawi* (Rodentia, Muridae). Environ. Eng. Sci. 2011; 28 (3):237-248.

[34] Kleiber M. The fire of life, an introduction to animal energetic: Wiley, New York. (1961) 454pp.

[35] Petter F, Lachiver F, Chekir R. Les adaptations des rongeurs Gerbillidés à la vie dans les régions arides. Bull Soc Bot Fr (1984) 131,

[36] Nagy K A and Costa DP. Water flux in animals : analysis of potential errors in the tritiated water method. Am. J. Physio. 1980; 238 :R454-R465.

[37] Banisadr G, Fontanges P, Haour F, Kitabgi P, Rostene W, Parsadaniantz SM. Neuroanatomical distribution of CXCR4 in adult rat brain and its localization in cholinergic and dopaminergic neurons. Eur J Neurosci 2002; 16:1661-1671.

[38] De Rouffignac C, Morel F . Etude comparée du renouvellement de l'eau chez quatre espèces de rongeurs, dont deux espèces d'habitat désertique. J Physiol Paris 1965 ; 58: 309-322.

[39] Nagy KA. Water economy of free-living desert animals. Int Cong series 2004; 1275: 291-297.

[40] Lacas-Gervais SG, Maurel D, Hubert F, Allevard AM, Doukary A, Maggi V, Siaud P, Gharib C, Sicard B, Calas A, Hardin-Pouzet H. Vasopressin and galanin expression in the hypothalamus of two African rodents, *Taterillus gracilis* and *Steatomys caurinus*, subjected to water-restriction. Gen. Comp. Endocrinol. 2003; 133: 132-145.

[41] Mbarek S, Saidi T , González-Costas J M, González-Romero E. and Ben Chaouacha Chekir R, Effects of dietary cadmium on osmoregulation mechanism and urine concentration mechanisms of the semi desert rodent *Meriones shawi, Journal of environmental monitoring* 2012 *accepted* DOI: 10.1039/C2EM30121K.

[42] Pettersen AJ, Andersen RA, Zachariassen K E. Effects of dietary intake of trace metals on tissue contents of sodium and calcium in mice (*Mus musculus*). Comp Biochem Physiol C 2002; 132:53-60.

[43] Wlostowski T, Karasowska A, Laszkiewicz-tiszczenko B. Dietary cadmium induces histopathological changes despite a sufficient metallothionein level in the liver and the Kidneys of the bank vole *Cletheriomys glareolus*. Comp Biochem Physiol C. 2000; 126:21-88.

[44] Leffel EK, Wolf C, Poklis A, White Jr. K L. Drinking water exposure to cadmium, an environmental contaminant, results in the exacerbation of autoimmune disease in the murine model. Toxicology 2003; 188: 233-250.

[45] Sudo J, Hayashi T, Kimura S, Kakuno K, Terui J, Takashima K, Soyama M. Mechanism of nephrotoxicity induced by repeated administration of cadmium chloride in rats. J Toxicol Environ Health. 1996; 48(4):333-348.

[46] Xu LC, Sun H, Wang SY, Song L, Chang HC, Wang XR. The roles of metallothionein on cadmium-induced testes damages in Sprague-Dawley rats. Environ Toxicol pharmacol 2005; 20: 83-87.

[47] Brzóska MM, Kamiński M, Supernak-Bobko D, Zwierz K, Moniuszko-Jakoniuk J. Changes in the structure and function of the kidney of rats chronically exposed to cadmium.I.Biochemical and histopathological studies. Arch Toxicol2003; 77: 344-352.

[48] Lynes MA, Zaffuto K, Unfricht DW, Marusov G, Jacqueline S, Samson J, Yin X The Physiological Roles of Extracellular Metallothionein. *Exp Biol Medicine* 2006; 231:1548-1554.

[49] Speakman J R. Doubly Labeled Water. Theory and Practice. London: Chapman and Hall- 1997. 416 pp.

[50] King JM, Bradshaw SD. Comparative water metabolism of Barrow Island macropodid marsupials: Hormonal *versus* behavioural-dependent mechanisms of body water conservation. Gen Comp Endocrinology 2008; 155, 2:378-385.

[51] Bozinovic F, Gallardo P, Visser GH, Cortes A. Seasonal acclimatization in water flux rate, urine osmolality and Kidney water channels in free-living degus: molecular mechanisms, physiological processes and ecological implication. J Exp Biol 2003; 206: 2959-2966.

[52] Wakerley JB, Poulain DA, Brown D. Comparison of firing patterns in oxytocin- and vasopressin-releasing neurones during progressive dehydration. Brain Res 1978;148 (2): 4425-4440.

[53] Arnauld E, Dufy B, Vincent JD. Hypothalamic supraoptic neurones: rates and patterns of action potential firing during water restriction in the unanaesthetized monkey. Brain Res 1975; 100 (2):315-325.

[54] Hiruma M, Ogawa K, TaniguchI K. Immunocytochemical and morphomometric studies on the effects of dehydration on vasopressin-secreting cells in the hypothalamus of the Mongolian gerbils. J Vet Med Sci 1992; 54 (5): 881-889.

[55] De Mota N, Reaux-Le Goazigo A, El Messari S, Chartrel N, Roesch D, Dujardin C, Kordon C, Vaudry H, Mosso F, LlOrens-cortes C. Apelin, a potent diuretic neuropeptide counteracting vasopressin actions through inhibition of vasopressin neuron activity and vasopressin release. Proc Natl Acad Sci 2004; 101(28):10464-10469.

[56] Callewaere C, Banisadr G, Desarménien MG, Desarménien MG, Mechighel P,Kitabgi, P, Rostène WH, Parsadaniantz SM. The chemokine SDF-1/CXCL12 modulates the firing pattern of vasopressin release through CXCR4. Neuroscience 2006; 103 (21):8221-8226.

[57] Callewaere C, Fernette B, Raison D, Mechighel P, Burlet A, Calas A, Kitabgi P, Melik Parsadaniantz S, Rostene W. Cellular and subcellular evidence for neuronal interaction between the chemokine stromal cell-derived factor-1/CXCL12 and vasopressin: regulation in the hypothalamo-neurohypophysial system of the Brattleboro rats. Endocrinology 2008; 149 (1): 310-319.

[58] Engelmann M, Ludwig M. The Activity of the Hypothalamo-Neurohypophysial System in Response to Acute Stressor Exposure: Neuroendocrine and Electrophysiological Observations. Stress 2004; 7 (2): 91-96.

[59] Antonio MT, Corpas L, Leret ML. Neurochemical changes in newborn rats brain after gestational cadmium and lead exposure. Toxicol let 1999, 104:1-9.

[60] Méndez-armenta M, Villeda-hernandez J, Barroso-moguel R, Nava-ruiz C, Jimenez-capdeville ME, Rios C. Brain regional lipid peroxidation and metallothionein levels of developing rats exposed to cadmium and dexamethasone. Toxicol Lett 2003; 144: 151-157.

[61] Gupta A, Gupta A, Shukla SG. Development of brain free radical scavenging system and lipid peroxidation under the influence of gestational and lactational cadmium exposure. Hum ExpToxicol 1995; 14:428-433.

[62] Ludwig M, Horn T, Callahan MF, Grosche A, Morris M, Landgraf R. Osmotic stimulation of the supraoptic nucleus: central and peripheral vasopressin release and blood pressure. Am J Physiol. 1994; 266 (3 Pt 1):E351-E356.

[63] Bundzikova J, Pirnik Z, Zelena D, Mikkelsen JD, Kiss A. Response of substances co-expressed in Hypothalamic magnocellular neurons to osmotic challenges in normal and brattleboro rats. Cell Mol Neurobiol 2008; 28 (8):1033-1047.

[64] Llorens-cortes C, Moos F. Opposite potentiality of hypothalamic coexpressed neuropeptides, apelin and vasopressin in maintaining body-fluid homeostasis. Prog Brain Res. 2008; 170: 559-570.

[65] Aguilera G, Lightman SI, kiss A. Regulation of the hypothalamic-pituitary-adrenal axis during water restriction. Endocrinology 1993; 132:241-248.

[66] Kregel KC, Strauss H, Unger T. Modulation of autonomic nervous system adjustments to heat stress by central ANGII receptor antagonism. Am J Physiol 1994; 266: R1985-R1991.

[67] Coburn CG, Gillard ER, Curras-Collazo M C. Dietary exposure to Aroclor 1254 alters centra and peripheral vasopressin release in response to dehydration in the rat. Toxicol. Sci. 84, 149.

[68] Kang JH, Jeong W, Park Y, Lee SY, Chung MW, Lim HK, Park IS, Choi K H, Chung SY, Kim DS, Park CS, Hwang O, Kim J. Aroclor 1254-induced cytotoxicity in catecholaminergic CATH a cells related to the inhibition of NO production. Toxicology 2002; 177:157–166.

[69] Sharma R, Kodavanti PR. *In vitro* effects of polychlorinated biphenyls and hydroxy metabolites on nitric oxide synthases in rat brain. Toxicol Appl Pharmacol 2002; 178: 127–136.

[70] Gillard ER, Coburn CG, Bauce LG, Pittman Q J, Curra′s- Collazo MC. Nitric oxide is required for vasopressin release in the supraoptic nucleus (SON) in response to both PACAP and dehydration. Program No. 660.1. 2004 Abstract Viewer/Itinerary Planner, Washington, DC: Society for Neuroscience, Online.

[71] Kadowaki K, Kishimoto J, Leng G, Emson PC. Up-regulation of nitric oxide synthase (NOS) gene expression together with NOS activity in the rat hypothalamo-hypophysial system after chronic salt loading: Evidence of a neuromodulatory role of nitric oxide in arginine vasopressin and oxytocin secretion. Endocrinology 1994; 134: 1011–1017.

[72] Donaldson, Z R, Young L J. Oxytocin, vasopressin, and the neurogenetics of sociality. Science 2008; 322: 900–904.

[73] Insel TR. The challenge of translation in social neuroscience: a review of oxytocin, vasopressin and affiliative behavior. *Neuron* 2010 ; 65 :768–779.